Testimonials

Having personally lost more than 100 pounds, I can tell you that Jackie understands what it takes to make a lasting physical transformation. With practical advice built upon strong spiritual underpinnings, she unravels the perplexing question of how to reach and maintain a healthy body.
—**Will Bowen, International Bestselling Author of** *Happy This Year* **and** *A Complaint Free World*

The reason I enjoyed your book is to put it simply -- it's a freedom to live an all-around balanced life! I think it was brilliant of you to have the sections so short. It made it really easy to just keep reading. This is a book that once you start, you just want to finish it and start doing what it says. I am now living Secret 7. I am loving life. There's no stopping me! — **God bless you!**
—**Renee**

The power of this story lies in its simplicity and its humanness. Ms. Trottmann has done a great job of communicating that there can be personal will and courage without fanfare. Her story telling is a refreshing and needed contribution to the literature on women's struggles: She experienced the emotional trials and pains of an eating disorder and she conquered them. A valuable and motivating read.
—**Terry Varney Freerks, Ph.D.**

I have struggled with my weight all of my life and for the first time I feel as if you have pointed me in the direction of The Truth and it is setting me free. I am following a Low Carb High Fat diet and was losing weight but was still a bit preoccupied with food. Not sure if I was eating from hunger or one of my many other reasons for eating. Then I read your inspirational book, The Freedom to Eat and listened to the meditation CD's. I have experienced a new level of freedom from all those unnecessary food thoughts. I eat so much less but feel so satisfied and am getting on with my life which is opening up again and I am one grateful woman. **So much of the battle was in my mind. Thank you so much!**

—**Kathleen**

I travel all over the world speaking to women about their passion and calling and unfortunately, I often find that many of them are suffering in secret. They are held captive and limited by pain from their past, struggles with weight loss, an attack on their confidence and identity. The message shared in this book is refreshing and provides real hope for women who desire to take back their freedom to eat and live life abundantly. Jackie's approach to this age-old struggle helps women go from suffering in secret to leveraging ten secrets to lasting weight loss and inner peace.

—**Lethia Owens, International Speaker and Founder of Audacious Faith – A Christ-Centered Community for Business Women**

*I never gave thought to the idea of eating just for the sake of food—letting food be food—until, through this book; I saw the simplicity of letting a meal be just a meal, not a substitute for the things I didn't want to face about my life. Now, I eat less, eat better, and enjoy my food in a different way. You are God's instrument for helping others find freedom by telling them about the path you are taking to find yours. It gives other people confidence in the guide and courage to read on.—**God bless!***

—**Louie**

Faith is a lifelong journey of growth and reflection. Through her words, Jackie has shared the journey of her life from deep pain to joy as she deals with a difficult childhood, weight issues, divorce and lack of self-esteem. I know this, because as one of her pastors, I have had the privilege to walk with her and witness her growth. Trusting in the God of love and mercy, she has reclaimed her life and found joy, meaning and purpose. May her words provide you with the wisdom and encouragement to do the same.

—**Rev. Dr. Karen Blanchard – Associate Pastor First Presbyterian Church of Kirkwood (St. Louis, Missouri)**

I'm loving your words so much because they are refreshingly honest and uncomplicated. – **Thank you!**

—**Loretta**

Since starting my personal training business over twenty years ago, I witnessed the struggle that women have with their weight and body image. After reading Jackie's book, I am somewhat in awe of how she has expressed that struggle so honestly and simply. I am proud of Jackie's fitness and professional achievements in the last ten years that I have known her. The Freedom to Eat is a great resource. I have already directed clients to this book to help them overcome their weight related issues.

—Rik Wilson, former NHL defenseman, personal trainer and fitness expert to clients from age 9-90.

The Freedom to EAT

10 Secrets for Lasting Weight Loss and Inner Peace

JACKIE TROTTMANN

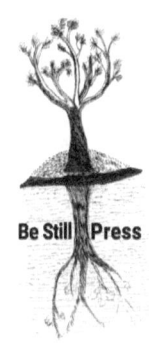

The Freedom to EAT
10 Secrets for Lasting Weight Loss and Inner Peace
Jackie Trottmann
Be Still Press

Published by Be Still Press, St. Louis, MO
Copyright ©2019 Jackie Trottmann
All rights reserved.

No part of this publication may be reproduced, stored in a retrieval system, or transmitted in any form or by any means, electronic, mechanical, photocopying, recording, scanning, or otherwise, except as permitted under Section 107 or 108 of the 1976 United States Copyright Act, without the prior written permission of the Publisher. Requests to the Publisher for permission should be addressed to Permissions Department, Jackie Trottmann. www.jackietrottmann.com/contact/.

All information contained within this book, is not intended to diagnose, treat, cure, or prevent any health problem—nor is it intended to replace the advice of a physician. No action should be taken solely on the contents of this book or website from which it was purchased. Always consult your physician or qualified health professional on any matters regarding your health or on any opinions expressed within this book or website.

Cover and Interior design: Davis Creative, DavisCreative.com

Library of Congress Cataloging-in-Publication Data

Names: Trottmann, Jackie, author.
Title: The freedom to EAT : 10 secrets for lasting weight loss and inner peace / Jackie Trottmann.
Description: St. Louis, MO : Be Still Press, [2018]
Identifiers: ISBN 9780998038902 (hardback) | ISBN 9780998038919 (paperback) | ISBN 9780998038926 (ebook)
Subjects: LCSH: Weight loss--Psychological aspects. | Food habits--Psychological aspects. | Self-perception. | Peace of mind. | BISAC: SELF-HELP / Eating Disorders & Body Image. | SELF-HELP / Spiritual. | HEALTH & FITNESS / Diet & Nutrition / Weight Loss.
Classification: LCC RM222.2 .T76 2018 (print) | LCC RM222.2 (ebook) | DDC 613.25--dc23

Library of Congress Control Number: 2018913572
2019

ATTENTION CORPORATIONS, UNIVERSITIES, COLLEGES, CHURCHES, EATING DISORDER CLINICS AND PROFESSIONAL ORGANIZATIONS: Quantity discounts are available on bulk purchases of this book for educational, gift purposes, or as premiums for increasing magazine subscriptions or renewals. Special books or book excerpts can also be created to fit specific needs. For information, please contact Be Still Press, support@JackieTrottmann.com

This book is dedicated to my husband who gives me the freedom to be me and who lets me know that I am completely loved; to my son whom I love to see grow every day; and to all those struggling with the physical, emotional, and spiritual weight that you carry. There is peace, love, forgiveness, and victory awaiting you.

Contents

Prologue | The Secrets We Keep xiii
Goodbye Diets—Hello Freedom 1
Stop the Needless Suffering 5
Part One – My Struggle 9
   Childhood Silencing the Still, Small Voice 11
   Food Became Love and Comfort – Let the Eating Begin 17
   Where Was God? 19
   Adolescence – Let the Comparison and Dieting Begin 21
   College – Looking for Love 23
   Enter the Voice of the Inner Critic 25
   Venturing into the World and
      Turning Away from My Faith 27
   The Demon in the Closet 29
   Desperately Seeking Any and Every Magic Diet Cure 31
   Having a Baby I'm Eating for Two! Three! Ten! 35
   Stuffing, and I Don't Mean Stove Top 39
   Five Words Changed Everything 43
   Awareness to the Rescue 47
   The Freedom to Eat and Much More 51
Part Two – The 10 Secrets 61
   Secret 1 – Awareness 63
   Secret 2 – Acceptance 73
   Secret 3 – Throw Away the Scale, Let Go of Judgments 83
   Secret 4 – Learn to Be Still, Let Go, and
      Trust by Practicing Meditation 97
   Secret 5 – Use Moderation, Listen to Your Body,
      Eat What You Crave 105

Secret 6 – Discover Who You Really Are,
   Discover Your Strengths and Talents 113
Secret 7 – Start Loving Life 123
Secret 8 – Invest in Yourself 129
Secret 9 – Clear Clutter from Your Life 135
Secret 10 – Make Life not About You Anymore 141
The Freedom to Eat 145
Epilogue 147
References 153
Resources 155
Acknowledgments 161
About the Author 163

Prologue

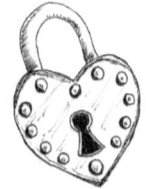

The Secrets We Keep

Like the Epilogue, this Prologue was written after the entire manuscript was finished. That's because everywhere I go, I meet new people and gain new insights (that is, after all, what Secret 1 is all about). It always amazes me what people share. Judging on outward appearances, I would never guess what is going on with people on the inside (Secret 3).

As a writer, I love words. The word *secrets*, used in the subtitle of this book, was chosen intentionally. That's because the definition of secret means: something that is meant to be unknown or unseen by others, concealed in such a way as to be accessible only to the person or persons concerned, something that is kept a secret.

What secrets do you have? If you struggle with your weight, your relationship with food, body image, self-criticism, doubt, fear, shame, self-loathing, and any number of other issues, I would venture to guess that you struggle in *secret*. The secrets to lasting weight loss and inner peace are hidden from you. You are too wrapped up in your present pre-occupation to see them.

This secret word came to life when talking with Patty. I was on a meditation retreat ending the old year and entering the new. Part of the retreat was silent. Ten years ago I would have called you crazy to ask me to participate in such an event! Now it's life-giving. Our favorite place to go is Timber Creek Retreat House, a non-profit organization run by founders and directors Beth and Tom Jacobs, not far from Kansas City. Robert and I try to go at least once a year. This was our fourth year. After walking on the trails, I stopped off at the kitchen and visited with Beth and Patty.

Patty is Tom's sister and is the chef. I had shared with Beth about *The Freedom to Eat* book. She mentioned the title to Patty and out came our stories... *secrets*.

Patty is beautiful inside and out. She has a twinkle in her eye and joy in her heart. The meals that she makes are amazing. They are a feast for the eyes, healthy, tasty and real food, nothing processed or out of a box. The house is always full of wonderful aromas from her latest creations. Guests will comment on Patty's joy, headphones plugged in, dancing as she chops and moves about the kitchen—her sanctuary.

During our visit, I learned that Patty had struggled with anorexia (her secret). She became chubby at around the age of eight or nine. Out of concern, her mother took her to their pediatrician. There were incidents of obesity in other family members, and they intervened before her weight got out of control. While it was humiliating enough to go to the doctor, she had to sit on the examination table in only her underwear. The male doctor looked at her almost-naked body assessing it for signs of puberty. Her mother was in the room, thankfully, but expressed no concern for the doctor's actions. This was in the early 1960's when doctors were looked upon as gods.

Patty couldn't help but feel humiliated and violated. She was put on a strict diet. And so began Patty's adversarial relationship with food and criticism of her body. Food became the enemy. Adding insult to injury, thanks to our model-thin, focused culture, Patty received lots of positive attention the thinner she became.

I was on the opposite spectrum, turning to bulimia as my final diet solution (my secret). My weight gain started around the age of thirteen. Food was the enemy for me, too. In Part I, I share my entire story of struggle and what finally set me free.

Our conversation lasted for quite a while and continued after the retreat as we shared our experiences. While different, there was a thread of obsession of trying to conform to an image that society presented to us as beauty. We were so blind that we couldn't see the beauty that was within us. All was outward, superficial, fleeting.

Patty loved to cook as a little girl. Her mother always encouraged her, but not as a career. Her parents were still afraid that the food would lead to obesity. Patty loves her parents and knows that her parents love her. Their intentions were meant to help not harm. It wasn't until just the last few years that Patty turned this passion into her livelihood. And what was shocking to me was that she had only stopped the extremely restrictive diets within the last eight months.

Paraphrasing from Amazing Grace, *we once were blind, but now we see.* We see the beauty of love, compassion, self-care, and creativity. We see that food is no longer the enemy. Food provides nourishment, pleasure, and represents community and fellowship when we share meals together. Food is not something that satisfies our need for control or that controls us.

We have set ourselves free and are at peace. It doesn't mean that we never have moments of self-criticism, but those are few and far between. We embrace our unique gifts and talents that we were given. For Patty it's cooking. For me it's writing.

I wanted to share this encounter because what we see and perceive will influence what we believe. On my travels talking about *The Freedom to Eat,* I encounter a lot of people who share the same struggle. It's not good to hold onto secrets.

If you are carrying a lot of emotional and spiritual weight, this weight can be much heavier than physical pounds reflected on a scale. Within these pages you will find relief. More importantly, you'll find the invitation to true freedom. By putting *these secrets* into practice, you will experience a lighter body, mind, and spirit.

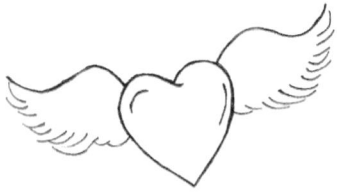

Goodbye Diets—Hello Freedom

If you are looking for the latest diet du jour, sorry, this book is not for you. If you are sick of diets, sick of obsessing about your body and every calorie, carb, and morsel you put in your mouth, read on.

Each year new diet books debut and become instant best sellers as people hunger for the magic cure to lose weight. Pun intended, hunger is what they continue to do. Eating is pleasurable, and dieting is painful! Of course, over-eating leaves its painful aftermath: self-loathing and never maintaining the weight lost for very long.

The Ecclesiastes author says, "There is nothing new under the sun." In the end, it is the quality and quantity of food consumption along with exercise that will achieve the goal of weight loss. Sure, some combination of foods or carbohydrates may work better for some than others, but to attain the ultimate goal, the Holy Grail of lasting weight loss, requires different thinking. In fact, it requires less thinking.

Dieting and obsessing about your body and appearance causes stress and anxiety. Overeating equally causes pain.

Thinking about what you are going to eat, counting calories or fats or carbs or protein clutters the mind. Added to the mind clutter are the self-criticisms: *I can't believe you ate that. You're a big, fat pig. You're pathetic.*

Then there are the false hopes that weight loss will bring like: *I'll be happy when I lose weight. I'll find the man of my dreams when I lose weight. I'll have more friends when I lose weight.* Fill in the blank.

When people are not happy and lose weight, especially when they reach their goal, there may be the short feeling of euphoria, but eventually, they will continue to be an unhappy person! Statistics show that the majority of dieters will gain their weight back and more. The problem lies in our attention focusing on the physical and listening to the wrong voices.

We listen to the latest diet gimmick, what the media, culture, teachers, religion, society, and even friends and family tell us to be, to have and how to look. Beauty is defined all around us and the examples are rarely anyone over the age of 30 (which makes matters worse if you're over 30). We stopped listening to the still, small voice within us. It's the voice that knows the truth. We've lost our connection to Spirit and sought answers outside of ourselves. We don't know that the Holy Grail we seek in lasting weight loss comes through a *holy connection.*

When we connect to our Creator and clear the clutter of obsessive thoughts that do not serve us, we are able to break free. If you have manufactured an image of God as an authoritative and judgmental male figure who is out there or up there and is as displeased and critical of you as you are (that's the God I used to know), you will be surprised to learn the truth. God wants to have a loving relationship with you and for you to live and thrive.

When we embrace an intimate relationship with a loving God, miracles happen. The miracles come in the form of lasting weight loss, overcoming obsessive, addictive and destructive behaviors, losing the "weight" of worry, doubt and fear, healing old wounds, experiencing many forms of forgiveness, and finding love and peace.

Freedom comes in living life in a spiritual flow. The hunger is gone, the physical hunger, the emotional hunger, and the spiritual hunger. We are able to eat (without starving or binging), to maintain a healthy weight, and return to the essence of our True Selves. It's tapping into and celebrating our glorious uniqueness. We look beyond the physical to discover and harness our talents to contribute to the world. That's *the freedom to eat.*

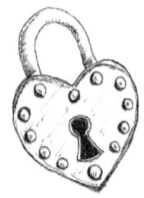

Stop the Needless Suffering

Meeting people for the first time at conferences or other events where *The Freedom to Eat* is the topic, I always tell people that I've lost over 500 pounds.

The reactions I receive range from huge smiles of admiration, or shock, to skepticism. Then I tell them it was the same 30 pounds over and over again. That usually draws a laugh. More often than not, people can relate to the struggle and frustration that comes with never achieving lasting weight loss. It doesn't matter if the goal is to lose five pounds or 500 pounds. In fact, I am amazed at the number of women I meet that say they need to lose weight. That's when *my* expression turns to shock because, in my eyes, they have no weight to lose. I shouldn't be surprised given my own struggle and the emails I receive from readers as they share that they are *not really overweight*, but have five or ten pounds they want to lose. (I call this bitten by the perfection bug. More about that later.)

Until I discovered what I call *the freedom to eat*, my mind was consumed with obsessive thoughts about food, my weight, and appearance. These thoughts possessed me like demons from the age of thirteen to forty-six. I have enjoyed *the freedom to eat* for sixteen wonderful years and counting. When I look back, I am amazed at the amount of wasted time, energy, and needless suffering that I caused myself.

Nearly every waking moment I was thinking about what I was going to eat that day. I judged my every action, constantly condemning myself for not looking like the models and movie stars. The scale was my judge and jury. It wasn't a fair one. If I had lost weight, I felt like I could cheat and eat something forbidden. If I gained weight, I berated myself and ate something forbidden with an attitude of, *what's the use?*

Now when I think of the words, '*cheat, forbidden, berate…*,' I realize how absurd it was to apply them to myself and my situation. Yet I lived my life in this self-imposed prison.

This thinking didn't happen overnight. It happened ever so slowly over time. This agony and suffering was the result of listening to the outside voices and not the voices of Truth. I had silenced my still, small voice starting as a little girl.

I mentioned briefly about the still, small voice within us. I believe that everyone has a still, small voice. It is a built-in guidance system that advises us and tells us what to do. Over the course of our lives, this voice molds us and shapes us into the people that we are. It is the voice of our soul, our true essence.

Those who are fortunate listen to this voice at an early age and heed its direction throughout their lives. For others, the voice is stepped on, stomped on, stuffed down, and ignored (many times through no fault of our own, as you'll see later) until it starts screaming to get your attention.

When I first wrote this chapter, I started writing about courage and how it took real courage to make a lasting change in my life. Then, I stopped to think about the words I had written. They didn't feel right. My words felt like a hollow motivational speech.

I realized that it wasn't so much that I had to *make a change* but that *I had changed* over time and had not even realized it. I had developed spiritual amnesia and had forgotten who I was. The real Jackie had checked out. I had stuffed down the real me and surrendered to the seduction of outside voices and images that we face every day: Look like this / Eat here / Drink this / Wear that. I had secretly started hating myself for not being able to conform to these outside demands. I use the word seduction because we are unaware of the effect all these images have on us at a deep, sub-conscious level.

Our culture fuels the problem, bombarding us with conflicting advertising messages. Not only does marketing glamorize unhealthy and/or excessive eating and drinking, they use beautiful, rail-thin models and actors to make their pitches.

What's funny and ironic about that last sentence is that the already rail-thin models aren't even thin enough. Thanks to advances in technology, the images are manipulated through further photo enhancement techniques. Every flaw and imperfection can be removed, and hips, thighs and buttocks can be whittled down with the click of a mouse. The role models we see are not even real. But we buy into the images.

There is another rub to this ideal image that we are supposed to live up to, and that is not to age in the process! Forty is the new thirty and fifty is the new forty we are told. Tell that to Mother Nature. In addition to being thin and wearing the right clothes, we are supposed to look like a thirty-year-old if we are fifty. How many ads are out there for anti-aging creams, gels, etc.? My husband laughs at the television ads and says, "Show us a sixty-year-old using the cream instead of a thirty-year-old!" There are injections, chemical peels and plastic surgery, too.

The message is loud and clear. **You are not good enough**. Sadly, we unknowingly buy into it completely.

Like many, I surrendered to these outside voices and images and had almost given up. What I needed to do was to succumb to a different kind of surrender. I needed to surrender to the fact that life was more than this. And in this case, surrender wouldn't mean giving up.

This type of surrender, which is discussed in recovery movements, means letting go of the behaviors and actions that no longer serve us. It is letting go of the struggle and turning it over to a Higher Power.

It's hard to listen to our still, small voice when all the other voices are not allowing it to be heard. It's also hard to trust our own voice when we can't trust those who are supposed to care for us or a Higher Power who is supposed to love us and not judge us. Here's how this struggle unfolded for me.

PART ONE

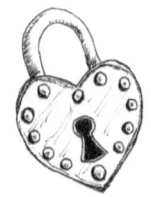

MY STRUGGLE

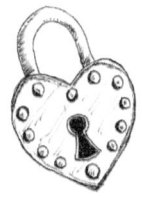

Childhood Silencing the Still, Small Voice

To understand why I silenced the still, small voice within me means to understand the events that silenced it. We all have signature events in our lives that influence our behavior whether they are positive or negative. Here are the events that would unknowingly impact my future.

As far as coming into this world, I was planned and welcomed. My older and only brother wanted a baby sister for Christmas. I didn't quite make it but came just three days later.

My parents met in World War II. My mother was from London, England. She met my father when he was stationed there in the Army Air Corps. Had the war not happened, my mother would have been a professional opera singer. Her singing genes were passed down to me and I could sing before I could talk. My mother still had her British accent. With her singing talent and smooth voice, it was like having Mary Poppins for my mother. She charmed (the r is silent - pronounced chahms) all that she met, and people would say, "Where are you from? I just love to hear you talk."

My father called me the *apple of his eye.* My mom and brother told me that I was Dad's favorite. When I was about four or five he used to take me to lots of Air Force parties and outings, just the two of us.

There were many children in our neighborhood and I had many playmates. There were no electronic games or thousands of cable channels to watch. We were expected to be out of the house and playing outside.

During this age of four or five, I was repeatedly molested by a neighbor while we kids would get together for games. I don't know how long of a time period this lasted, because I didn't know what was happening or what to do. This was my first lesson in silencing my still, small voice and discovering the power of denial. Each event I would block out. I never told anyone because I didn't know how.

My father worked as a security guard for a large brewery. His hours involved working the evening shift. One of my fondest memories was a tradition we had on Saturday nights. My brother and I would stay up late and watch the monster movies. I'd be scared to death watching The Mummy or The Werewolf, or another classic horror movie. Then my father would walk through the door carrying a bag of tamales that he purchased from a street vendor as a late-night snack for us to share. We would unwrap our tamale presents from their corn husk wrapping, slather them with ketchup, and then eat them as we watched the end of the movie together. I remember how safe I felt and how unafraid I was because my daddy was home. It was an idyllic time.

Several years later, things started to change on the home front. Part of the perks for working for the brewery was getting to drink all the fresh beer that you wanted. My father took full advantage of this perk. His drinking became severe and with the drinking came a change in his behavior. There were no more outings. There was no more love or support from him. I felt confused and abandoned.

Alcohol affects people in many different ways. Some people become the life of the party, while others become angry and violent. Because of alcohol's power to lower inhibitions, I believe that what lies deep within a person will manifest their true behavior. Unfortunately, in my father's case, the alcohol brought out all the anger he felt inside.

He would come home from work, rant and rave, and then pass out into a dead sleep. Then he would go to work the next day. While he was not physically abusive to *me*, he was physically abusive to my mother.

Nowhere to Hide

Our house was a small, five-room ranch that consisted of two bedrooms, a kitchen, living room, and one bathroom. With only two bedrooms, my brother had his own room and I slept out in the living room on a fold-out sofa. Every inch of space had to be used effectively and efficiently.

There was a pantry in the kitchen the size of a small closet. On the inside of the door, from top to bottom, hung every cooking utensil, pot, pan, and knife we owned. In addition to my mother's wonderful singing voice, she was a fabulous cook.

During my father's boisterous rants, there was nowhere to hide. On this particular day, Dad was extremely angry; about what, I don't know. He cornered my mother in the kitchen and began to slam her up against the inside of the pantry door.

I watched her back hit all the sharp, metal objects as he continued his assault. I couldn't believe he was doing this. On a deep, subconscious level, my thoughts were, *No one treats my mom this way!* I had become possessive of her at that moment.

With all of the strength that a twelve-year-old little girl could muster I screamed, "Stop it! You're hurting her!" It took every fiber of my being because none of us confronted him. I had watched long enough and had summoned all of my courage which came out of me like a roar.

It worked because he stopped and immediately turned and looked at me with such hatred and hissed, "Then I'll come after you." All the courage vanished as I cowered, backing out of the kitchen to escape.

My distraction, however, had saved my mother and had allowed her to instantly call the police. They arrived very quickly.

I breathed a sigh of relief thinking that the police would take this horrible man away. We would tell them what happened and we would be safe. They would see how mean he was and would lock him up.

The police came inside, and my father's demeanor transformed from a crazed Jack Nicholson in *The Shining* to Mr. Rogers. He crooned to the officers that everything was fine. The policeman bought the act! I couldn't believe it! He was even telling jokes with them by the time they left.

The next day when my father went to work, my mother changed the locks on the house. We were safe for a while.

With changing the locks, my mother's next plan was to try to leave. My father went into a rehab facility to get off the alcohol. Since my mother didn't work outside the home, she had no source of income. When she talked to a lawyer and to the Welfare Department to get financial aid, they told her that she would have to give me up. Well, that wasn't an option. It was really a low point for all of us. I emotionally shut down and couldn't leave the house. I developed agoraphobia—an irrational fear of public or open spaces. At that time, I had a very active social life at school and especially with my youth group at church. However, I was so gripped with fear and anxiety that I wouldn't and couldn't leave the house. I missed a full week of school during seventh grade.

There weren't any other options. My mother had no alternative other than to take him back. I remember tears running down my face when my father came into the bedroom and said, "I want to come home." I said, "I don't want you to come back," as he hugged me. He was on his best behavior for a while. I forced myself to go back to school.

There was some comfort in growing up, however, and that was with my closest friends. Their fathers were also alcoholics. I remember being at Stephanie's house and her father would be screaming. I thought, *wow, this is just like at home.* The same thing happened at Toni's house. Her father's veins would stick out from the sides of his neck and his face would turn beat red with his tirades. It helped to confirm that my life was somewhat normal. At the same time, however, I always thought, *there's got to be something better than this.*

Upon my father's return, my goal during those trying years was to get out of the house as much as possible. The violent outbursts came and went, and no one said anything about them. It was very confusing. Whatever feelings were there were stuffed down, never to be shared. Denial became my closest friend.

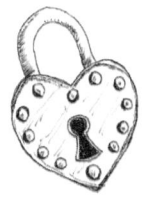

Food Became Love and Comfort – Let the Eating Begin

At the same time, I was dealing with the new challenges and emotions brought on by puberty. Lacking the support and attention that I craved and not knowing how to deal with these feelings, I turned to food for love and comfort to fill that void.

There were lots of confectioneries around our school that served sandwiches and snacks. Even though I had lunch money, it wasn't enough to fill my insatiable appetite. When my father would pass out after one of his rants, I would tip toe into my parent's dark bedroom and go into his coin purse that was on the night stand. I remember my heart pounding as I tried not to make a sound. Then I would steal several quarters out of his coin purse. The entire time I was terrified that he would wake up and find me stealing. He never did, so I continued this ritual to support my food habit.

As a result of my overeating, I started to gain weight. My clothes weren't fitting anymore. Food, my only comfort, had turned on me, too.

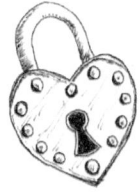

Where Was God?

My father was Catholic and my mother was, as she described herself, "A broad-minded Baptist." As what happens so many times, the mother can be the spiritual leader in a household. In our household, Mom took us to church, the Lindell Boulevard Bible Church.

Church played a big role in my life growing up. Being involved in choir and with the youth group provided a sanctuary away from the dysfunctional environment at home. Unfortunately, the image and teachings I learned about God at church were equally dysfunctional. The message from the pulpit was that I was a miserable sinner. God was not a loving heavenly Father but a judgmental and vengeful heavenly Father that was waiting to, as I like to say, "squish me like a bug," if I stepped out of line.

It was bad enough that I had an angry earthly father. Going to church and learning of God's nature left little comfort. Rather than have Bible verses highlighted with love, compassion, and forgiveness, all the Bible verses I had highlighted were of laziness, gluttony, or a litany of many other shortcomings to confirm my unworthiness.

One of my favorite ones was Proverbs 23:2, "And put a knife to thy throat, if thou be a man given to appetite." Or Proverbs 23:21, "The glutton will come to poverty." I even dated the latter verse in the margin of my Bible, February 13, 1971. (Pretty inspirational, don't you think?)

This added insult to injury in turning to God for comfort. My prayers were filled with groveling and very little gratitude.

Still, I sang and worshipped and believed in God. For certain, I always tried to *please* God; in fact, I tried to please everyone. But I knew, deep down, with God I never measured up.

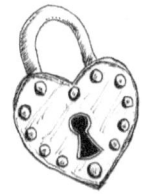

Adolescence – Let the Comparison and Dieting Begin

As a teenage girl, I started reading all the teen magazines. I suddenly became conscious of my clothing size and compared myself to others. What it summed up for me was that I wasn't good enough. I had to be better. I became anxious about my weight. For me, anxiousness translated into eating more. My weight started to become an issue. The solution to this problem, of course, was to go on a diet. Drastic measures were required, so drastic diets were the answer.

This is when the thirty years of diet madness began.

There was the protein diet, the Scarsdale Diet, then the Atkins diet. I gained five pounds on Atkins. I thought I could eat all the fried pork rinds I wanted. Then there were diet pills. My mother would let me have one of her diet pills when I was particularly upset. In the 1960's, these were amphetamines. One pill would keep me awake for two days. I even resorted to wrapping my entire body with plastic wrap, donning sweat pants and a sweat shirt, and sitting up in our attic during a St. Louis killer, hot summer day to try to do something instantly. This was not an attic where there were stairs to pull down. I had to carry a six-foot step ladder from the basement, climb it and pop a three-foot by three-foot portion of heavy wood and plaster out of the ceiling to gain access to the attic. This can be called being highly motivated, desperate, or silly! Like everyone, I was looking for a quick fix. It worked. I dropped a few pounds of water, but gained it back as soon as I drank any liquid shortly thereafter.

The Internet wasn't around back in the early 60's offering endless promises of instant results by ordering the latest supplement or exercise contraption. I would have hounded my mother for money to purchase it all.

The first diet sodas came on the market in the early 60's. The taste of the initial artificial sweeteners was dreadful! But they were like manna from heaven because they didn't have any calories. I remember eating dill pickles when I drank one to wipe out the aftertaste.

It's no wonder that I didn't develop any boundaries toward eating. I had no boundaries for anything. At home I felt like I was walking on eggshells every day not knowing what side of Dad would show up.

He left the family after one last stay in the detox ward. At that time, I was graduating from high school. When he was living with us we just thought alcohol was the problem. He was later diagnosed with bi-polar disorder. Unfortunately, during the fifties, sixties, and even the seventies, mental health was not as sophisticated a science as it is today. There is a better understanding of neurological disorders and resources are available to receive help.

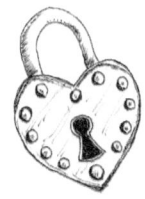

College – Looking for Love

I hated high school and doubled up on my classes so that I could graduate early. No one was giving me financial support to go to college, so I went to work immediately after graduation to save money. As soon as I had enough money saved up, I left my home in St. Louis to attend the Moody Bible Institute in Chicago. Because of my love for singing, I decided to be a voice major. My short-term dream had been to join a college choir and go on tour. I had that opportunity with the women's glee club.

At this point in my life food was still an issue; however, the school experience was exciting, so eating didn't consume all of my thoughts. Also, having picked a Christian college, I was surrounded by a much-needed safe and nurturing environment.

Secretly, my long-term goal in attending a Christian college was the hope of getting my M-R-S (Mrs.) Degree. Even with the terrible role model of my father, I still believed in fairy tales and that true love existed. I had chosen the Moody Bible Institute because of my strong faith and what better place to meet Mr. Right?

In my freshman year, I fell in love with a senior. During our time together we were inseparable. He was from Manitoba, Canada. Talk about geographically undesirable! After he graduated we wrote each other a few times. There was no email back then and long-distance phone calls were extremely expensive. The relationship faded away quickly. It was a painful loss. I felt abandoned once again by a man that I loved.

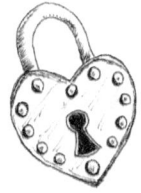

Enter the Voice of the Inner Critic

This voice is different from the still, small voice that leads us and guides us. The inner critic is our false voice, but its presence is so insidious that we listen and follow its commands. If we let it, our critic will smother the still, small voice of Truth within us. The inner critic can be so powerful and so persistent that we don't even question it.

This is the voice we hear that tells us we are not good enough, or we doubt and criticize ourselves. My inner critic raised its ugly voice and told me that I wasn't going to make a career of singing. I needed to go home and do something more practical. So, I made the decision to return home.

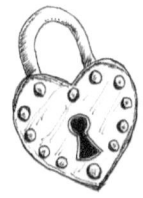

Venturing into the World and Turning Away from My Faith

I had no friends. They had all graduated, married or moved away. I lived in isolation. The only job I was able to find was as a typist for a huge accounting firm. Life consisted of going to work, returning home, and watching television. My mother had always struggled with her weight too, so we joined a weight loss program together.

I would always reach a point in my weight and clothing size when the pleasure of eating didn't outweigh the pain of how I felt. I guess I did have some boundaries buried away after all!

All of this was magnified by my social isolation and the fact that I was, once again, living in my parent's house. I was working at a pay-by-the-hour job for an amount just over the minimum wage in a dreary environment.

I'll never forget my twenty-first birthday… a milestone. I celebrated it alone in my car in the parking lot of a fast-food restaurant. After that incident, I didn't feel that something had to change; I felt that everything had to change!

I loved art, music, and business, so I decided to quit my job and return to school to earn a business degree. I also attended church for the first time in ages (I had given up that, too). On the way home, I purchased a newspaper and was thrilled to find that a local advertising agency was looking for a part-time receptionist. The field of advertising had all the characteristics that interested me in a career. The ad said to call Denise. I called her the next day and got the job. Things were looking up.

That phone call ended up turning into a career in marketing and sales that lasted over 30 years. Denise and I are still friends. Another huge bonus that resulted from that one little phone call was meeting the man who would become my husband. Having a successful career and a happy marriage was great!

When I met my husband, I quit going to church. I turned away from my faith completely. Life was working out quite well without God's help. In fact, I found it quite extraordinary that I hadn't been "squished like a bug." The only problem I had was the ongoing struggle with my weight.

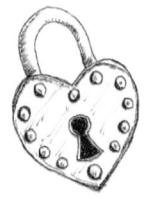

The Demon in the Closet

My closets were full of various clothing sizes including the one skirt, or pair of pants—something which was two sizes too small that I would find on sale and buy. The tiny garment was meant to provide motivation.

With zippers and buttons bulging in a dressing room, I would look at myself in the mirror with a combination of disdain and hope. With the gusto of Scarlet O'Hara and her famous, "I'll never go hungry again," I would look in the mirror with hope and silently scream, *I'll never be this fat again!*

The garment would hang in my closet with the tags still attached. Instead of providing the desired motivation, this demon would sneer the words, "Ha! You're a failure!"

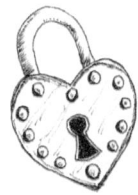

Desperately Seeking Any and Every Magic Diet Cure

B y the time I was in my late twenties, the weight loss industry had grown to offer many promises of quick fixes and magic cures. When my pain became unbearable, I joined one of the pre-packaged providers. This was great! I didn't have to think except about how little I was going to eat and when. But that was okay because they provided everything!

Okay, that worked for a while. But I liked wine and margaritas. They didn't have any pre-packaged alcoholic beverages.

By now, the teen magazines had been replaced with the latest and greatest fashion magazines. In addition to the current role models being beautiful, they were all wearing and/or were surrounded by very high-ticket merchandise. Now I was comparing myself to women who were rich **and** thin. The competition had stepped up because the bodies were getting more glorious and the material possessions were added to the mix.

These magazines had frequent articles about bulimia and anorexia. I certainly couldn't relate to anorexia as I couldn't imagine not eating anything; however, bulimia really piqued my interest. Clearly, the idea of eating all that I wanted then purging was an ingenious idea. In fact, just the word *purging* was perfect. By literal definition the word means: *to purify, to make free of something unwanted—to clear of guilt*. Certainly, after binging on huge amounts of food, purifying myself seemed almost a holy act. My indiscretion of consuming too many calories could immediately be undone.

I tried it after indulging on margaritas and chips. I had too many margaritas anyway, which made the process very easy. Wow, this was great! I had found my answer to eating and drinking whatever I wanted on Friday and Saturday nights.

This was working out so well that I started doing it on weeknights, too. I rationalized that I didn't do it every day, so it was okay.

One day, I noticed that I had begun to form a callus on my middle right finger. I thought, *huh, that's weird*. Then I realized the callus was a result of sticking my finger down my throat repeatedly.

The tragedy in this situation lies in one glorious word—purging. If the articles had said that bulimia is binging and then vomiting, I'm not so sure I would have embraced the idea. After all, who in their right mind would want to vomit on purpose?

The word 'vomit' still brings back every ghastly memory I had of the flu or food poisoning. I remember a time as an adolescent at camp. The meatloaf turned out to be bad. One by one, each camper had that overwhelming feeling of nausea. It was a feeling of helplessness knowing that it was coming and there was no way to stop it. We mentally prepared to face running to the bathroom to be violently sick.

Great spiritual and philosophical teachers will tell you that the mind is the key to controlling how we view ourselves and the world.

In my mind, I had found an answer to a problem with my binging and that was the beautiful act of purging. At this time in my life, I was in my thirties. Bulimia was supposed to be a practice done by young people. In another twisted way of thinking, I considered myself to be young and caring about my looks and appearance like a teen or twenty-year old. That was how delusional and desperate I was in my mind.

The helpful fashion magazines dutifully reported the problem of tooth enamel erosion that plagues many bulimics. So, I was very careful to rinse my mouth after every episode of purging. But there was one problem with this system, I wasn't losing any weight. Eventually, I started to feel that this wasn't such a great idea, but I kept doing it anyway. Thank God, I was saved from this terrible cycle by…. my baby. I became pregnant.

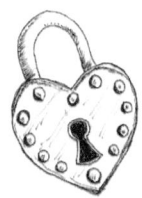

Having a Baby
I'm Eating for Two! Three! Ten!

Looking back, I must say that I have adopted some positive health habits. I have always been a fairly healthy eater. Fresh fruit, vegetables, fish, and chicken have been staples in my diet. I've never been one to gorge on potato chips, french fries, or fried foods. I also have been somewhat of an athlete and exercise has always been a passion for me. So, inactivity was never an issue.

My problem was two-fold; I had an all-or-nothing attitude about food and I was unconscious of my eating. Cereal, pizza, and ice cream were some of my favorite foods. In reasonable portion sizes, these foods can all have a place in a healthy eating plan. The pleasure that went along with eating these foods, however, was too great because I never stopped with a healthy portion size. I would eat an entire medium Domino's pizza at one sitting. Standing, watching television with only a handful of my favorite, healthy cereal, turned into my unconsciously eating half of the box. A perfectly measured half cup of ice cream turned into two, three, four servings then sometimes led to half the container.

In my head were a set of rules of what I could and couldn't eat. The rules were all or nothing—on a diet or off a diet. I was either perfect or a loser. I didn't eat what I *wanted* to eat. I ate what I was *supposed* to eat, according to the latest diet of the week. The end result; I was never satisfied. I would keep eating until I ate what I wanted in the first place.

Let me give an example of my absurd, internal dialogue:

I would really like a piece of that apple pie.

You can't have a piece of apple pie, it's fattening. It has 350 calories.

Yeah, you're right; I'll have some cottage cheese and pineapple. That's only 300 calories and it's healthy calories.

Yes, good.

There was only one problem, I still wanted the pie. This dialogue would go on and on as I continued to eat healthier, calorie-laden alternatives and eventually would eat the pie too. The overeating made me furious towards myself. This is what crazy, obsessive thinking looks like.

When I became pregnant, I immediately stopped drinking alcohol and other beverages that were potentially unhealthy for my baby. The withdrawal from my morning caffeinated coffee resulted in three weeks of headaches and lethargy. But the purpose was worth the pain. I was determined to take care of my growing child; unfortunately, I grew right along with him!

In some respects, being pregnant was liberating for me because I couldn't diet. I *had* to eat. It was my first experience of being free to eat anything I wanted and as much as I wanted (which is different from *the freedom to eat*). I set an all-time personal weight record of 210 pounds. Of course, I didn't care because I assumed I would lose the weight after this fifty-pound baby was born. Oh, wait, babies only weigh about 10 or 11 pounds maximum. I was certain that I was carrying a 10-pound baby and a 40-pound placenta.

Another way that being pregnant was liberating for me was that the obsessive thoughts about my weight and my body stopped. For instance, the fact that I had no ankles anymore didn't bother me. My legs had turned into limbs which were straight up and down from my knees to my feet. I had never stopped to appreciate that I had defined ankles before. They were still there. I just couldn't see them at the moment. I had a mission and a purpose much greater. That mission was doing everything possible to ensure the outcome of having a healthy baby.

The General Manager at the radio station where I worked had her last child. She was very generous and gave me all of her maternity clothes. The majority of these clothes were beautiful Laura Ashley jumpers. The yards of fabric concealed my sixty-pound weight gain and then some. I could have had triplets with room to spare. Wearing these jumpers made me feel beautiful. She had purchased so many that I never had to worry about what I was going to wear. That was freeing.

As I approached the 210-pound mark, the absurdity of my own body image finally came to light. I was rearranging my clothes closet. My yo-yoing in weight throughout the last ten years resulted in having sizes of tens when I was heavier and eights when I was getting skinny. I continued to have my one or two pieces of clothing with the tags still hanging on them meant to inspire me to lose weight once and for all. There were many more size ten items. Some designers are kinder than others, so I purchased the roomier size tens. If I had to move up to a twelve, I wouldn't buy it.

I came across a very cute, size ten, black cocktail dress, with spaghetti straps and a sheer, flowing skirt. With the dress still on the hanger, I held it in front of me to admire. I hadn't been able to see my feet without the benefit of a mirror for quite some time, so I was admiring my dress from a considerable distance while thinking, *how in the world could you have ever thought that you were fat? You couldn't even get one leg into this dress now. Wow....*

My baby boy arrived, weighing seven pounds thirteen ounces. I can guarantee you that the placenta didn't weigh forty pounds. Thankfully, I had retained a tremendous amount of water and lost most of that weight in the first two weeks after his birth; however, I still had about twenty-five pounds to go.

The baby's arrival was the greatest accomplishment of my life; unfortunately, this wasn't the case for my marriage.

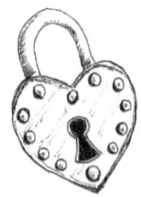

Stuffing, and
I Don't Mean Stove Top

My husband and I worked in the advertising business. It was very easy for our jobs to be all-consuming. At the time, I didn't realize how we had begun to live separate lives. Becoming pregnant brought us closer together. At least, that's what I thought.

I remember when I first told people that I was pregnant; they would repeatedly say to me, "Your life is going to change forever." Perhaps my habit of practicing denial dismissed this recurring message. I thought this was an odd thing for people to say. But changing from a couple to a family brought out problems that were brewing underneath the surface of the marriage.

This event, did indeed, change my life. My career had been so important to me, but all I could think about was staying home with my son. That wasn't an option. I took another job that promised more flexibility. It didn't. My husband took a promotion in another state. We planned to move. My entire world was turned upside down.

Had my mother not been there to help take care of my son for me when I went back to work, I don't know what I would have done. Here I was with a new baby and it was supposed to be the happiest time of my life. All the care I had taken, all of my hopes and dreams I'd imagined for this event had turned into a nightmare. All I wanted to do was to get things back to "normal."

We put our house on the market, but the promotion he had so desired wasn't the job he wanted. Thankfully, he was able to step back into his prior position. My previous employer welcomed me back with open arms. We did sell our house, but moved into a dream home in a neighborhood much closer to where we both worked. I stuffed all of my feelings down. We went on about our lives, now with our son.

Denial, busyness, and shear willpower can be powerful friends when we don't want to face our feelings. I summoned all of them. With stepping back into our prior jobs, this stopped the pain. All was back to the "normal" I was seeking.

Some people eat when they are depressed. Others lose interest in food. I guess it's a blessing that I lose interest in food. I was certainly depressed during this time. But my son was my primary concern and he was a huge source of joy. My obsessive thoughts about food were gone.

Having eaten to my heart's content during the pregnancy, I settled down for about a year. Food didn't hold the same fascination. It's funny when you can have anything you want, you suddenly don't want it so badly. Once the tumult of the prior months subsided, however, I went back to old eating patterns. Food was a source of comfort. Alcohol was my drug of choice to feel good and change my emotional state. Unlike my father, alcohol made me happy.

Stuffing, and I Don't Mean Stove Top

I would hit my high weight and life would become very painful for me. The solution would be to join a different weight loss plan.

I was constantly gaining and losing. If I counted up the pounds over the years, they would have been more than the 500 that I stated earlier. It was always the same fifteen to thirty pounds.

All this madness stopped one day when my choir director said five words to me.

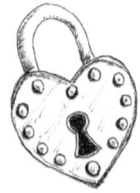

Five Words Changed Everything

Writing this, it seems hard to believe I had abandoned my singing for almost twelve years and my faith for twenty years. When my son was seven years old, my still, small voice was beginning to speak to me to find a church where we could attend as a family. I started the process of shopping churches and found a new church home in our neighborhood, First Presbyterian Church of Kirkwood, Missouri.

Four years later, we acquired a new Director of Music who expressed an enthusiastic interest in working with me with one-on-one voice lessons. He was a young, animated German and an extremely talented musician and teacher.

We were in his small office and the door was closed while I was taking a voice lesson. The piano was facing the wall which meant that his back was facing me as he sat playing scales or a piece of music. I stood behind him and sang, following his instructions.

Suddenly, he stopped playing and in a sweeping motion, he swung his legs around on the piano bench, planted his feet on the floor, faced me and in an exasperated voice barked, "Why won't you let go!"

The words startled me and had the effect of a bucket of cold ice water being thrown in my face. Deep down, I knew why I wasn't letting go.

The life I had was not the life I wanted. My entire life had been built on what I *should* be doing. I had stuffed my feelings and buried my heart, soul, and entire being with busyness, material possessions, food, and denial.

My son was now eleven years old. Those five words released all the hurtful feelings and emotional pain that I had suppressed since the traumatic period shortly following his birth. Although I had always loved the life I have had with my son, I finally faced the reality that I was going through the motions in my life and my marriage.

The Rat Wheel

I describe my life at that time as the rat wheel. Every morning I got up at 5:30 A.M. to be the first to use the only full bathroom that we had in the house. I then got my son ready, would drop him off at school and head off to work. At the end of every work day, I would pick up my son and head home to make dinner and help with homework. On a good day, I had the opportunity to take a walk with my dog. At the end of the day, I would put my son to bed and then fall into bed exhausted, only to repeat this routine day after day after day.

The irony of the situation was that we had two pet rats! We actually owned a rat wheel which our rats ran on every day. The difference between their wheel and mine was that they ran for fun and all of their needs were being met. Their rat wheel was the good life.

My wheel never stopped moving from sunrise to bed time. I was running as fast as I could to stay on the wheel and getting nowhere but exhausted in the process.

The busyness saved me from thinking. The material possessions and successful career provided me with self-esteem and showed the world that I was meeting the requirements of living the American dream. Food was my drug of choice to bring me pleasure and comfort. Denial was wrapped nicely around this entire package, not allowing my heart and soul to feel and know the truth. The truth be told—I was lost.

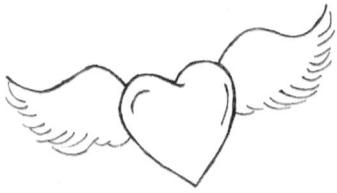

Awareness to the Rescue

My emotional pain had become overwhelming and I knew that I had to do something about it. I couldn't just leave my marriage, even though I was hurting. I didn't want to hurt my husband or my son.

To cope through the stress, I decided to try some yoga videos that I had received as gifts. The instructions emphasized the importance of not forcing the moves, treating yourself gently, listening to your body, and breathing to relax.

Wow, treating myself gently? That was a unique idea. I was always striving and beating myself up. I immediately fell in love with this process. The practice helped me de-stress. I began to pay attention to my body. At the end of the exercise, I felt completely relaxed. My life did not feel out of control anymore.

I had never learned to be still. As a result, an amazing thing happened. I became aware of being hungry or more importantly, not being hungry. This was a first. I had never missed a meal. Before I started yoga, it was my habit to eat at every mealtime. If it was breakfast time, it was time to eat. If it was lunch time, it was time to eat.

Once I started this practice I noticed that there would be days when noon would roll around and I wasn't hungry, so I didn't eat. Then one o'clock would come around and I would be hungry. I am embarrassed to say that with all the hunger in the world, I never truly felt hunger. I was starting to become aware of my body and I was starting to *feel*.

The yoga began to quiet my mind and I began to become more aware of everything. That's when my choir director's question came back to me, "Why won't you let go?"

I did finally let go one day when all of my suppressed emotions and feelings bubbled to the surface. I realized that I had been using food to numb myself and in the process stuff my feelings. I stuffed them down so far that I didn't know how to feel.

I truly believe that when we are ready to receive, people appear to help us. At work I had started confiding in someone about my feelings, my past, and my marriage. This co-worker asked me if I had ever heard of co-dependency. I had no idea what she was talking about. She recommended a book called *Co-Dependent No More*.

I went to the bookstore, picked it up and began to thumb through the pages. It talked about people with alcohol addictions and drug addictions and how their behavior affects all the people around them. Co-dependent people had the characteristics of feeling guilty, becoming a workaholic, overeating, having a lot of "shoulds" in their life, expecting to do everything perfectly, not having fun, and being afraid to let themselves be who they are.

I was dumbfounded that this book talked all about *me*! I purchased it immediately.

There is a phrase that I've started using in many circumstances in my life, "I didn't know what I didn't know." Until I read this book,

I didn't know the true impact that my father's behavior had had on my life. I dismissed this past and stuffed it away never dealing with the consequences. I truly thought alcohol and his behavior was **his** problem, not **my** problem.

I repressed any needs that I had because I simply didn't know how to express myself, period. I had no role models to show me how to express myself. If I cried when I was little, my mother would soothe me and tell me, "Now, now don't cry." She never cried. One had to be strong. She wasn't being mean. This was her way of coping that she passed down to me. So, I would rarely cry and never cry in front of anyone.

Once I began to understand myself and how I had emotionally shut down for so many years, I found the courage to tell my husband that I couldn't go on in the marriage. It was extremely hard to make this announcement and it was a long process, but I was finally being true to myself.

The fifteen to thirty pounds that I struggled with all of my life just melted away. Part of that was due to the trauma of the divorce and leaving the marriage. I was extremely concerned about the negative impact that this would have on my husband and my son. My body was in an overdrive state. I could feel my metabolism speeding up as a result. The daily yoga was also changing my form. I went from a size ten to a size four. At one point I felt I was too thin. Those are words that I never thought in a million years that I would say.

Once I moved out of our home, the divorce was in progress and I came to the conclusion that my ex-husband and son were going to be fine, my body settled into its new normal. The extra weight has never returned. I've stopped obsessing about my weight, dieting, and found my voice.

One of the great things I did was to leave the scale behind. I never plan to own a scale ever again. (I'll explain about the power the scale had over me in the Letting Go of Judgements Secret.) The only time I step on a scale is when I go to the doctor's office. It's funny because the scale still has somewhat of a hold on me. If I weigh more than what I was expecting, I watch more closely what I am eating. However, if it's what I was expecting or less, I tend to indulge for a while.

I monitor how I feel and also how my clothes fit. I can sense when I've been indulging too much. For me, that means I've been eating too many carbohydrates like bread and butter when I'm out at dinner or indulging in desserts. If I drink alcoholic beverages, I have one and savor it. I no longer use alcohol to change my state or numb pain. The pain has been replaced with inner peace.

I'm aware of what I'm eating, so if I indulge, I simply watch what I eat a little more closely in the days ahead, focusing on eating more fresh vegetables and lean protein. And I always step up the exercise. Simply stated, I continue to listen to my body. That means that I eat when I'm hungry and I stop when I'm full. This is no longer a foreign concept but a way of life.

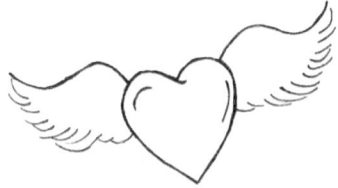

The Freedom to Eat and Much More

Letting go of old hurts and pains from my past has allowed me to love myself and, in turn, allowed me to love and be loved by others.

In my prior marriage, I missed the most important part of my life: my faith and close relationship with God. I had abandoned my connection with God completely. My focus had been solely on my mind and body and nothing on my spirit. I was seeking approval from everyone and felt empty. I did not bring a whole person to the marriage, but I brought a lot of emotional baggage that I had never addressed.

I have remarried. My husband, Robert, and I met at church. Our getting together was definitely through divine intervention!

Through our friendship, we learned how we shared similar life experiences during our prior marriages. Through our love, we discovered that we are, in every sense of the word, soul mates. Our love is based on our love for God. Faith is our foundation. I love him for the wonderful person that he is, and he loves me completely. Our marriage is a true partnership.

For over a decade, I trained with a personal trainer, Rik Wilson, twice a week. My father-in-law had given me a check for Christmas one year and I decided to use it to see a personal trainer. I had no idea that I would be continuing for this long. Initially, my goal was to build strength and distinct muscle form. I had already been at my ideal weight for four years.

The results have amazed me. Not only have I gained strength, but also self-confidence and stamina. While I have led a fairly active and athletic life, I have never been in better physical shape than I am now. I have walked my dog for miles at a time, three to five times a week, but did not practice strength training, until I met Rik. Our workouts had become more than that. He had been a source of inspiration and support as I've struggled with ups and downs in my professional life. As I get older, I've also realized the importance of strength training for holding on to bone density, especially for women.

Robert was a marathon runner and competed in many bicycle races. We spent some of our early dates riding our bikes on local trails. Prior to my initial training sessions with Rik, I was exhausted after riding for five or ten miles. I felt a big difference between riding a bike and walking. By working out with Rik, I continued to build my muscle strength, and now, I can complete a twenty-mile bike ride with lots of energy to spare. My daily walk up and down the stairs in our house is now an effortless task. I find myself standing taller and straighter for long periods of time without feeling fatigued. These are just a few of the many little things which add up in making a big difference in my life.

For fifteen years I have maintained a size four-six figure. I mention it because for me, this size is beyond any goal I had set for myself. I never dreamed that I would be wearing a size four anything. When I was a teenager, I went as high as a size fourteen. My body has settled at this new size.

Everyone's body type is different. The way that clothing fits us is different. My wedding dress was a size eight. So, I mention the size because we all have a healthy baseline weight that is right for us.

Losing this weight made a dramatic difference physically in my health statistics like cholesterol numbers and mentally in my well-being.

On occasion I'll read a fashion magazine when I am at the salon or spa. I noticed that the new, ideal fashion sizes are now size zero and two! The stakes just seem to get higher in the new goal for beauty. I have no desire to be a size zero or two. If I did get to a size zero, my bra size would be a zero! So, the goal is to be healthy and happy.

I am encouraged to see that some advertisers are showing images of various, realistic body types. Even *Sports Illustrated* has depicted curvier models on their swimsuit covers. Times are changing. That's a good thing.

For the past decade I've discovered the power of meditation. I, again, reached a point of busyness in my work life. Though I no longer struggled with my weight, I noticed joy slipping away from my life. I had somehow surrounded myself with toxic work relationships. It turns out that co-dependency lingered in this area of my life also. Just as I had introduced yoga into my life, I started meditating and learning to be still, first for ten minutes, then twenty minutes a day. Choosing to include meditation and other contemplative practices into my daily routine has changed my life for the better. I'm so passionate about meditation that I created a series of meditation CD/s/MP3s: *Be Still, Let it Go, and Trust.* The Let it Go CD/MP3s is the companion to this book. Each meditation corresponds with the 10 Secrets. Learn more at JackieTrottmann.com.

Meditation clears clutter from the mind. Through this new clarity, I identified another area of my life that I wanted to transform, and that was physical clutter.

When I married Robert in 2004, it marked my second move within two years. My first move was from a large four-bedroom home into a very small two-bedroom home. The majority of my things were packed in boxes and found their home in the new basement. The second move brought me and all my boxes into Robert's home, where we share a little more space. And again, the boxes made their way into the only space that was available—the basement.

Moving is one of the most stressful events in life. Nothing goes as planned and issues tend to pop up. How do you move a queen-sized bed up a narrow staircase into a small home that was built before there was such a thing as a queen-sized bed? What happened to the bolts needed to reattach the refrigerator door? And how can I make sure the cat doesn't freak out and run out of the house at the first opportunity?— just to name a few!

None of the boxes were sufficiently labeled or marked, so the movers deposited them wherever there was room. The result was a disorganized, cluttered nightmare. There wasn't even a path to walk through the piles of boxes. The good news was that this mess was *only* in the basement, and we had a great solution: close the door.

Fast forward, four years after the move: I quit my job in corporate America to pursue a full-time consulting career, which meant I worked out of our home. I knew the ancient art of Feng Shui involved decluttering by designating a place for everything. I also read that the layout of the rooms in the house was important to bring about positive energy; however, I needed additional assistance to bring order to this mess. There was someone I had met years ago at a women's networking function, so I sent her an email requesting a consultation.

I received a phone call from Samantha Shields, a Feng Shui expert. She came over and gave our home a thorough evaluation. What I learned was incredible. Just as I learned about pushing down my feelings and how I used food to assist in that manner, I learned why I used clutter to hold onto limiting beliefs, especially as it pertained to finding my life's purpose.

I told Samantha that I felt "stuck" and the basement and its clutter felt like a weight on me. She shared that with Feng Shui, the basement represents the past. By clearing out the basement, I would be clearing out old memories, habits, relationships, thought patterns, etc. She then proceeded to say that when we are stuck and can't find the time and effort to declutter, it can be due to a number of reasons. Maybe we think we will use an item again, or perhaps we have an emotional attachment to the person who gifted the item, or perhaps there are attachments we don't fully understand. Whatever the reason may be, when we declutter, we are choosing to let go of life connections from our past.

She gave me an action plan to carry out over the next few weeks. Time went by and I did minimal work. I found myself shuffling things from one box to another. Samantha pointed out that there was something else going on and that I was holding onto the past. With quite an indignant tone, I responded to her statement with, "I don't care about anything in the basement or the past." To which she asked, "Why don't you just get a dumpster?" I was silent for a moment and then I said, "Good point."

I'd felt completely overwhelmed by the mess in the basement and the task of clearing it out. Samantha worked with me to go through sections at a time and gave me tasks that made an immediate difference, such as moving things around to create floor space. As I began to throw out broken and useless items, I started to feel lighter. I found two wardrobe boxes full of clothes from my heavier times. It was fun to try them on and see that not only did the clothes not fit me, but that the style didn't represent who I was anymore. I took most of the items to my church for distribution to women that are in need of work clothes and the rest went to Goodwill. Clearing up the space immediately made my heart and mind clearer.

I mentioned that when we are receptive, the right people show up. Not only did Samantha show up to help me, but a friend had just returned to St. Louis, after losing everything while trying to establish her career in New York. She was literally homeless and had sold all of her possessions. Another friend owned a vacant house and had recently taken it off the market. She agreed to allow my friend to live there temporarily. Since Robert and I merged our households, we had almost two of everything. The timing couldn't have been better for my friend or us. I invited her to our basement to go shopping. She took a bed, lamps, desks, cookware and many other items. It was wonderful to be able to provide for her through our unused possessions.

Everything in our world contains energy. Yoga and meditation made me slow down and become conscious of my body and spirit. This consciousness spilled over into all areas of my life. It is why the basement went from being a place I literally shut off to a place where

I began placing all of my attention and recognizing the effect of the clutter.

My basement was stacked with old files from prior jobs, old bills, papers, old books filled with concepts and beliefs I no longer held, clothes from a prior life, failed business ventures, and on and on. Now that was bad energy!

This energy permeated throughout the house, in smaller doses as well. While I would not consider myself a slob, I would never consider myself a neat nick either. The clutter in the kitchen or my office would pile up and then I would spring into action to straighten it all up. I have since found this process exhausting and also just another sign of low self-esteem. Our homes are a reflection of who we are, along with our cars, purses, wallets, etc. If they are a mess, that is a sign that something deeper is going on.

It took a concerted effort to clear out the basement so that it was no longer a weight on my psyche. There were many trips to Goodwill, various other charities, and the public library. When I dropped off a box of books at the library, I told the librarian that I was clearing clutter from my life. She replied, "It's like you are getting wings, isn't it?"

Walking out of the library that day with my empty boxes, I thought about what she said. With a big grin on my face and a joy-filled spirit, I thought, "Yes, I do feel like I have wings!"

Just as my heart had been closed, by ignoring my feelings, I remembered I had dreams which I'd put away deep in my mind. I was living in the shadow of other peoples' success and had buried my dreams. One dream was to be an artist.

While I am not currently pursuing a career in art, I felt an overwhelming desire to draw and paint. One day, my husband asked me what I wanted for my birthday. I immediately shared that I saw a box of artist pastels, watercolors, and pencils that I truly desired. After I received the gift, I visited an art store to purchase some drawing books and brushes to go with them. I spent a long time browsing through all the various art supplies, and chatting with the helpful people about the items I needed and how I was excited to create art again.

I paid for my items and then walked to my car. I got in and suddenly began to cry uncontrollably. I felt like a little child again. All through childhood and until I graduated from high school, I was obsessed with drawing and painting. Then, the voice of my inner critic reared its ugly head to tell me that I wasn't good enough to be Norman Rockwell. So, just like that, I stopped drawing, just like I had stopped singing. My tears were a release from past judgments and the joy of returning to something I so loved.

If I could go back in time and talk to that senior graduating from high school, I would have told her, "Of course you're not Norman Rockwell silly, you're YOU."

When searching for designs to include at the chapter headings, my editor said, "Why don't you draw them?" So, I did! I also added the cartoons.

Another gift I received from meditation was the realization that I have always wanted to be a writer. Clearing the clutter from the basement helped me to clear the way for new opportunities in my life. It also gave me the courage to act. I found a journal from 1977 and discovered my writings focused on getting control of clutter and my desire to be a writer. That was decades ago!

I'm finally pursuing that dream full-time. The first draft of this book was written in a beautiful area I created in the basement.

I've since written another book: *God Notes – Daily Doses of Divine Encouragement*. (Visit JackieTrottmann.com to find out more.)

My mind and soul are free from the constant chatter. As far as food goes, I eat whatever I want, whenever I want. I don't count every calorie or fat gram that goes into my mouth. And there are many days that I'm not interested in eating because I don't know what I have a taste for. That is a miracle to me because before, all I could think about was food and my love/hate relationship with it.

Gone are those days of hate. I hated parties because I felt fat or ate too much. I hated the way I felt if I overate. I hated feeling too full. Today, holidays and vacations are a joy! I no longer have to worry about gaining five or ten pounds during these events. While I may eat unhealthier food during this time, I don't eat past the point of feeling full. If I happen to go overboard, I make sure that I am mindful of making healthier choices for my indulgences or I simply step up my exercise routine.

My father-in-law was amazed at the amount of food I ate when we would get together. He would say, "Look, she's a member of the clean plate club." Part of the reason that I can eat so much is because my body is healthy now. I've not starved it into slowing down my metabolism through low caloric intake. I'm also not yo-yoing back and forth, gaining and losing ten pounds constantly. Through my weight training, I have built up muscle mass and muscle burns more calories than fat.

I'm still not perfect by air-brushed, model standards. Who really is? I am strong, healthy, and filled with peace. Gone are the multiple wardrobes. When I buy any new clothes, it's usually because my other clothes might be dated or worn out!

When the seasons change, it still amazes me when I put on an outfit that I haven't worn in a year and it fits. When I get ready for a party, I don't look in the mirror and think, *does this make me look fat,* or criticize every body part. I have let go of all past hurts and have found my heart.

Every New Year, losing weight is not on the New Year's resolutions list. In fact, I no longer have New Year's resolutions. Instead, I cherish each day, move in the direction of my dreams, and am open to opportunities that come my way.

Life is too short to be consumed with thoughts that take away your joy and purpose. It is like being locked in an awful prison. The only limits in life we set are self-imposed.

The following chapters outline the ten secrets that helped me transform my life and continue to bring me the lasting weight loss and inner peace I know today. It would bring me the greatest joy if I could help you unlock what is holding you back and what is keeping you from your freedom.

Think of these secrets as a treasure hunt. You are searching for buried treasure. That treasure is uncovering and discovering the ultimate, unique, and incredible YOU.

PART TWO

THE 10 SECRETS

Secret 1

Awareness

These secrets are spiritual principles, touchstones to living a life with peace, joy, lightness, and personal power. As I mentioned in the Prologue, I call these secrets because they were hidden from me. I discovered the power of each principle on my journey to *the freedom to eat*. That's because I finally listened to the still, small voice within. You have this power within you when you choose to pay attention to what's inside and stop listening to the outside voices.

Awareness is not only a powerful secret for weight loss; it is a powerful spiritual principle for life. Awareness is the unshakable foundation on which all the secrets build upon each other. The first secret towards *the freedom to eat* is recognizing or being aware that you have behaviors that are not serving you well. I am referring to destructive behaviors that cause you to ignore your feelings, your body, and your thoughts. Change cannot begin until you acknowledge that you need to make a change. This change means returning to the ultimate and wonderful you.

Awareness also means being conscious. Did you ever drive someplace and then forgot how you got there? Driving can become an automatic act as you detach your mind from driving and your actions take over. When you drive to a familiar place, your body instinctively pushes the gas pedal to move forward and turns the steering wheel in the direction you want to go. Some of your behaviors may have become so automatic that you are totally unaware of what you are doing.

So, you must identify these behaviors. I've included some questions to help you explore your various behaviors. This is not a time to judge yourself, but a time to be aware and truthful. Jesus said, "You will know the truth, and the truth will set you free." It's important to note that some of these behaviors may be so ingrained and set in your unconscious mind that you may have to dig deep. These behaviors may also be painful to admit.

Just like the yoga videos instructed me to be gentle with myself, this is a time to be gentle with yourself. This is a time devoted to self-nurturing and self-care. It will not be easy to feel pain. But it's important to feel the pain then let it go.

Think of awareness as being an unattached observer. You are like a scientist in a lab looking through a microscope just observing behavior with no judgments. Think of my phrase, "I didn't know what I didn't know." As you start to become aware, you will find yourself saying, "I didn't know I did that!" **When you recognize these behaviors, you can change them.**

1. **Do you constantly think about food or what you are going to eat for your next meal?**
2. **Are you a binge eater, meaning, do you eat large quantities of food at one sitting?**

3. Do you sneak food?

Are you even aware of it?

Are you hiding this even from yourself?

Let me give you several examples of what I mean by sneaking food. There's a birthday party at work and everyone gets together to have the celebration in the lunch room, chats, and has cake and ice cream. The rush of sugar kicks in and you want more, but there's no way you are going to take another piece of cake in front of everyone. If you did that, everyone would know that you have no self-control and that's why you're overweight. The cake is left in the lunchroom and when no one is looking, you go back and grab another piece and eat it secretly.

Or, you're making dinner. I love to cook and it's important to taste what you are cooking to make sure the seasonings are just right. Tasting can sometimes turn into eating a complete portion size unconsciously. Most likely, no one is looking when you are cooking. In a warped sense, the mind rationalizes that because someone doesn't see you eating, the calories don't count!

Leftovers can be a huge issue. I remember many times shooing off the people to help me clean up as I cleaned other family members' plates. This wasn't cleaning with just soap and water. I'd eat the leftover crust of garlic bread, meatloaf, mashed potatoes, etc. Then there were the last of the leftovers in the pots and pans that I would eat.

This is kind of a funny story on sneaking food. One time my husband caught me eating out of the ice cream container standing at the kitchen counter with my back to him. He was laughing because my elbows were tightly tucked in against my body like I was trying to be invisible. He wasn't judging me at all. He just found the pose to be funny. At that moment I too laughed at how I must have looked.

Unfortunately, instead of learning from that experience that *eating ice cream was okay*, I made sure I wasn't *caught* the next time.

4. **Do you have bad eating habits such as starving yourself all day and eating an extra-large meal later in the evening, or worse, eating all evening?** Consuming all of your calories in the evening has three consequences: 1) you'll most likely eat more because you rationalize that you haven't eaten all day, not to mention that you feel like you are starving, 2) eating all of your calories late at night, without any exercise, doesn't allow the opportunity to burn off those calories, and 3) eating all of your calories at night is robbing your body of the fuel and nutrients it needs throughout the day for you to function at your best. Remember, food represents the needed nutrients and fuel for your body first and foremost. (I forget that sometimes too.)

5. **Are you aware of what you eat, when you eat, or are you distracted while eating?** This includes being in *auto-pilot* mode, in front of the television, or in the car while eating an entire bag of potato chips or fat-free snacks.

One day, I came home early from the radio station, around four o'clock in the afternoon. It was a rare occasion, plus, I had the house to myself. My favorite wine at that time was white Zinfandel. The Oprah Show was on the air and I decided to treat myself to a glass of wine with some cheese, fruit, and crackers while I nestled in a comfortable chair to watch the show. I didn't stick to one glass. Within the hour, I had drunk the entire bottle of wine! I was, frankly, shocked that I had drunk the entire bottle of wine by myself.

Not wanting to raise suspicions with my husband for the missing wine, I covered up the bottle in the trash can and went to the store to replace it. That never happened again, but even that incident didn't bring my awareness to the issues I had with food and the shame it produced.

6. **Do you taste and savor your food?**

I mentioned in my story of struggle that my mother was a fabulous cook. I am so grateful that she was a culinary master long before Food Network. Thanks to her inspiration, I love to cook. It's only been since I've had *the freedom to eat* that I truly taste and savor food. One of my favorite things to do is to try to identify the ingredients in dishes and enjoy the smell, feel, and texture of food. There is nothing like a perfectly ripe strawberry, nectarine, or melon. The smell is like perfume and the burst of flavor that comes from a perfect piece of fruit is luscious. I grow my own herbs and there is nothing better than cutting off some fresh thyme or rosemary and sticking my nose in the middle of a bouquet. The fragrance is as intoxicating as smelling a perfect rose. There's no guilt in eating something so naturally fresh and nutritious.

Guilt comes when we assign good and bad to the food we are eating. This will be covered more in Secret 5. Of course, we should strive to eat a healthy diet full of fresh food, few processed foods, or unhealthy fat and calorie laden foods.

While on the retreat I mentioned in the Prologue, we spent twenty-four hours in silence. It started one evening after dinner and lasted up until dinner the following evening. There were ten of us that attended the retreat, and we all ate three meals together.

There is always lively conversation going on at meal-time. During the silent portion of the retreat, however, we ate our meals in silence. That act brought to my awareness how quickly I tend to eat my food. This was not an entirely new awareness. That's because I am married to one of the slowest eaters on the planet. Robert has always chewed his food slowly. I have made a conscious effort to slow down so that I'm not sitting in front of him with an empty plate! But during the silent dining, I became very mindful of my eating. Chef Patty, makes incredible, healthy food, and I chewed and chewed enjoying and savoring each bite. Since that time, I have slowed down in my eating to enjoy and savor each bite. I confess, I used to do this only during a lavish meal or indulging in some decadent dessert. Now I'm putting this mindful eating into practice.

Not every meal will be a culinary blockbuster, but strive to eat tasty food. Food should not only provide us nourishment; it should engage all the senses.

7. **Do you eat while driving or eat while working at your desk?**
8. **Do you find that you eat a lot of sugar or lots of high carbohydrate foods, such as white bread and pasta?** These foods are metabolized quickly, making you feel hungry faster. We are all individuals and some foods affect people differently. A high sugar diet can cause people to gain weight and to almost have an allergic reaction to some foods. Medical research shows that high sugar-type foods, especially sugar-laden drinks such as regular soda, fruit drinks, fruit punches, energy drinks, sports drinks, sweet tea, and other such sugary drinks can lead to type 2 diabetes.
9. **Do you eat a very low fat or no fat diet?** The low fat and no fat craze has created a lot of high carbohydrate products that may be low fat but laden with sugar (read the labels). No fat also doesn't mean no calories.

Eating a reasonable amount of fat will help you feel full and eliminate cravings for more food. Certain fats like olive oil, walnuts, almonds, and avocados contain healthy fats.

10. **Read labels.** Starting in 2017, the FDA made restaurant chains with 20 or more locations list calorie counts and additional health information upon request. According to the USDA, the average number of calories for a woman to consume each day is between 1,600-2,400 depending on how active you are. For men, it's between 2,000-3,000 each day. While I don't mention counting calories, it's important to have awareness of the nutritious value of food.

On a recent visit to a popular chain, I was shocked to see how many calories were in the food! Robert and my son didn't appreciate my reading every calorie listed out loud, but I couldn't help myself: "A full rack of ribs: 2,388 calories, turkey burger: 1,312 calories, french fries: 728 calories, sweet potato fries: 935 calories!" The fat content ranged from 270 grams (out of 280 total calories for salad dressing) to 1,182 grams for the ribs. Various research shows that fat intake should be between 44-78 grams a day. So, you can see how not being aware of what is in your food can not only sabotage your efforts but be dangerous to your health!

11. **Do you eat when you're happy, sad, lonely, bored, angry, and anxious? Do you eat for any reason other than being hungry?**
12. **Are you anorexic or bulimic?**

If these questions don't ignite feelings within you, then sit quietly and think of behaviors that are causing problems for you. In some cases, you may need to seek professional help, especially if you are suffering from Anorexia or Bulimia.

It's important to take as much time as needed to explore these questions. You can begin to become more aware of your behaviors and discover what is *eating you* and why you are not happy in your present state. Start a journal and write down the questions that seemed to spark some pain or discomfort.

Some readers may find it difficult to connect to their feelings. If this describes you, the reason lies in not putting yourself first. Women, especially, are caretakers. We take great pride in taking care of other people and ignoring our own needs. In one word it comes down to love. We lack love for ourselves. We may have spent years (for me it was decades) denying our true feelings. I don't know why but somewhere along the way we bought into the notion that loving ourselves is a selfish act. Don't hesitate to ask for divine guidance.

In the Gospel of Mark, a teacher of the law asked Jesus what commandment was the most important. He replied, "Love the Lord your God with all your heart and with all your soul and with all your mind and with all your strength." The second is this: "Love our neighbor as yourself. There is no commandment greater than these."

The key here is loving your neighbor as yourself. Loving yourself is equal. If we don't take care of ourselves with rest and sleep and healthy eating, we have nothing to give. Decades of denying our feelings may not bring them to the surface overnight. Keep writing, getting quiet, and asking for spiritual guidance until you feel you have released any painful emotions. One of my favorite prayers is, *Help*. To help you embrace each spiritual secret, I've included a special prayer at the end of each chapter. There is a companion Let it Go CD that features these prayers to meditative music. You can listen to each meditation for each secret. This will help you to replace your disempowering thoughts with empowering thoughts.

Here's a note I received from Nikki:

Jackie! Thank you for your Let It Go CD. It is helping me rewire my mind into more positive thoughts and feelings about myself. The more I listen to it, the more it helps me de-stress and become the renewed child of God I would like to become.

The affirmations are very short and are set to meditative music. You can purchase the Let it Go MP3s or CD here (the CD has a little prayer book inside) at JackieTrottmann.com.

There are two additional meditation MP3s or CDs: Be Still and Trust. You can learn more about all three at JackieTrottmann.com

Remember, the purpose of this first secret is to acknowledge the truth about your behaviors so you can move forward into *the freedom to eat*. The added bonus is that practicing awareness will open yourself up to any number of opportunities for growth by shedding destructive habits and beliefs.

A Prayer for Awareness

Dear God,

In the noise and busyness of life, I thank you that my body is quietly supporting me.

Help me to practice awareness in all areas of my life.

Help me to be aware of your presence in my life and in the world.

Each day I become more aware of my body and spirit.

I am aware of the world around me.

I am aware of the tone of my voice—how I talk to others and how I treat others.

I am aware of how I talk to myself and treat myself.

Thank you for your perfect love. Because of this love, I treat myself and others with loving kindness.

Thank you for this wonderful body.

Help me to be aware of how everything I eat and drink affects my health and well-being.

I am aware of getting the proper rest and exercise.

I am aware of how much better I feel emotionally and physically—when I get the proper rest—move my body—and eat well.

My awareness helps me to listen to the still, small voice inside of me.

My still, small voice leads me and guides me in all areas of my life.

My awareness lets me pause and observe every situation.

Through your power and presence within me, I can handle any challenge without reacting.

I respond in a positive way.

Help me to bring this quiet peacefulness and awareness to my day.

Amen

Secret 2

Acceptance

I have found acceptance to be one of the most simple and powerful spiritual lessons to learn. Once you recognize your behaviors, you can then start to accept how those behaviors caused specific issues in your life. This is a time for self-discovery and gentle self-care. You may have developed behaviors that resulted from poor choices, causing potential weight and health issues. What caused these behaviors was not your fault. Most of us used eating as an unhealthy way to fill our needs that were not being met.

I want to focus on the prior sentence—What caused these behaviors was not your fault. I don't want this sentence to mean a lack of personal responsibility. In my search for wholeness, I saw these very words in one of the many books or articles I read. To become aware that my father's aggressive behavior wasn't my fault was freeing. As a little girl, I had no guidance or support to deal with his outbursts. As a result, I internalized it all feeling guilty and blaming myself for somehow causing his behavior.

Children many times will blame themselves for their parents' divorce or conflicts. Many abused children grow up to become abusers. Alcoholic or drug addictive parents can produce children with the same addictions.

For years I took great pride in breaking our family's cycle of alcoholism, and physical and verbal abuse. My father's behavior was so unacceptable to me. I couldn't understand how anyone could treat another human being that way. I also couldn't understand the need to be addicted to alcohol or drugs.

Truth be told, *I didn't break the cycle*. True: I had not become an alcoholic. True: I didn't physically and verbally abuse others. *True: I became my own victim of abuse by using food and hateful words as my weapons, thus, continuing the abuse cycle. I **had** become an addict. I was addicted to food and to work.* Remember, "The truth will set you free."

You don't have to have grown up in an alcoholic household to have feelings of unworthiness or abandonment. Many children have parents who are extremely successful and pillars of the community. They provide their children with a stable home life and unlimited opportunities. Materially, children may be cared for, but emotionally they may equally feel abandoned. If fathers and mothers have not received nurturing, they feel that their part is that of provider. They run their households like they run their positions in the office. Perfect parents expect perfect children leading by example but not emotionally connecting. The child's material and physical needs are met, but emotionally they may feel bankrupt. This causes as much confusion for a child as an abusive relationship.

Whatever your situation, simply accept that it is what it is. Feel the unfairness, the hurt, and the pain, and then let it go. Accept the way you reacted and coped and let that go, too. Now that you have accepted your behaviors, you can change internally so that food becomes fuel to live, something you enjoy that brings pleasure into your life and not pain. Food serves your need for nourishment and sustenance, when you choose not to give it control over you.

I am a proponent of keeping a journal. Even as a teen, I found time to write. The act of writing connects us closer to our hearts and draws out our true feelings as we put them on paper. In my twenties I had abandoned core values and activities that were the foundation of my being growing up: my faith, drawing, and singing. My advertising career had taken all of my focus. When I met my husband to be, he read one of my journals without my knowledge or permission. After finding that out, I felt betrayed. My journals have always represented the private window to my soul. In my all-or-nothing way of dealing with issues and confrontation, I simply stopped writing. It wasn't until ten years later, when my son was born, that I wrote again.

As in the past, when I had no one to turn to, I turned to my journal. I will never abandon writing again.

The divorce changed how I journal completely. Instead of chronicling events, and writing about feelings on the surface, I search for answers within myself. The answers always come as I dig deeper. Instead of questioning the choices I have made, I look deeper into why I've made my choices.

Once on paper, you can see your behaviors and search your heart for reasons for your actions. This is not a time to judge, but a time to understand who you are and what has shaped you.

Don't let the idea of writing be intimidating. Remember, writing is an opportunity to be honest about your feelings. Open and honest writing is not concerned about proper sentence structure or grammar. It may feel like writing as a first grader. (Sometimes that first grader in you may need to be heard, too.) It's quite okay.

One way I use writing is as an on-going healing process. When you write about feelings, be honest. Write at least two full pages, ideally three pages and let your thoughts flow. This may be hard at first, but keep writing. It may not be pretty. The purpose is to write and to express your inner feelings. Let all the hurtful words, and wounded feelings fly. There may be many. This style of writing brings out your ugly critic.

I know this seems like a contradiction when I mentioned that this is not a judging exercise. Unfortunately, we tend to be very judgmental. (That's why Letting Go of Judgments is Secret Number 3.) The fiercest critic we have is ourselves. You must draw out this ugly, *lying* critic and expose it. Only then can you silence it. Silencing your critic takes practice, but over time, this ugly monster can turn into a distant voice that you will be able to dismiss simply by telling it to be still.

The reason I said ideally three pages is that something magical happens after you've ranted for the first two pages. You start to receive insights. You aren't buying the critic at face value. You start to question and say, "Hey, that's not true." I can't explain how this happens. It just does. The only way to believe me is to try it.

Remember, easy does it. Stop saying hateful things, thinking hateful things. Many times, the way we treat ourselves internally can be horrible! Could you imagine saying those words to anyone else? Yet we may say the most awful things to ourselves. When you catch yourself saying these words and being critical, you must simply stop.

Secret 2 – Acceptance

Practice walking past a mirror saying "I am a child of God." Then, "No one else is like me." Look into the mirror and say out loud, "You are loved." And then, "I'm living my best life now."

If you feel harmed by others, write a letter expressing how you feel. I wouldn't recommend sending the letter. What is important is that you are expressing your feelings and your thoughts. This is about expressing your own feelings, and not condemning others. You are getting it out so that you can let it go.

Many times the last person we are willing to forgive is ourselves. If you haven't experienced awareness in your life, chances are the people that have hurt you or are hurting you will not be aware of the hurt they are causing you or others. They may *never* become aware. What's important is to not let *their* actions or *your* actions hurt you any longer. Ask God to help you to move past your hurt. When you hold onto resentments and judgments, it is like poison. You want the other person to suffer; yet, unknowingly; *you* are the one that suffers. You become stuck. Replaying the tapes of past hurts and resentments over and over again will keep you from living your life and moving forward. You must let it all go.

God made every one of us. Just as no two snowflakes are alike, no two people are alike. The Psalmist said, "For it was You who formed my inward parts; You knit me together in my mother's womb. I praise You, for I am fearfully and wonderfully made." Believe it.

You are here for a reason and that reason is to experience love, forgiveness, and joy each day, and to remember and rediscover who you really are.

God created you with an internal guidance system and that system is your feelings and instincts. When you are in touch with your feelings, you know what to do. When you are not in touch with them, it's usually because you just stopped listening to this guidance system.

Accept that this is an on-going process. This is not a diet program. It's about losing the physical and emotional weight that you carry. This is about living the life that you dreamed possible, because you will have freed your mind of all the clutter of thoughts that no longer serve you. You've freed up your heart to receive and give love. You no longer hunger and feel empty. You have been restored to wholeness, how you were initially created, whole.

True Healing Power

Though these steps came from my personal experience, the result of confiding in others and writing down personal feelings have been documented by many research studies. I completed two fifty-hour courses through Stephen Ministry and Stephen Leadership at my church. Stephen Ministers and Leaders are lay people who are trained to offer Christ-like care. During the classes I learned about Professor James W. Pennebaker, Ph.D. He is the author or editor of 10 books and almost 300 scientific articles and ranks among the most-cited researchers in psychology, psychiatry, and the social sciences. I reached out to him and was thrilled that he allowed me to share this research taken from his book called *Opening Up: The Healing Power of Confiding in Others*. The book was based on an ongoing study from 1977-1990 with his graduate students at Stanford University and Southern Methodist University in the area of mind/body relationships and health. Among the strong indications of the research were:

- Personal disclosure, opening up, is beneficial to health and recovery from illness
- Suppressing deep guilt/turmoil requires arduous physical effort and is devastating to health
- Confiding in a journal, spouse, or friend profoundly and physically relieves stress
- It's not the size of the trauma but our level of self-disclosure that determines our well being
- Inhibition affects short-term biological changes and affects long-term health as a cumulative stressor on body and mind
- Writing is always safe, no one will judge you, criticize you or distort your perceptions—BUT—there's no feedback
- Sometimes it is necessary to have a professional listener: counselor, minister, therapist
- Choose a confidant carefully—the listener must be accepting of the speaker

The more you can get in touch with your true feelings, the easier life will become. When you work through the hurts and pains, you will be free to live in the present moment. While you can't change your past, once you practice acceptance, you can then let the hurtful past go.

Acceptance is an on-going spiritual practice that will serve you. Why? Because life is about change. The Greek philosopher, Heraclitus, is known for the quote: "The only thing that is constant is change." Change can be good, and change can be bad. We can accept change or suffer by not accepting it. But change will happen.

All of us are aging. With aging comes change. That can mean loss: loss of health, loss of wrinkle-free skin, loss of abilities such as driving, mobility, and energy. Losing loved ones, treasured pets, and treasured friends.

This is not to depress you, but to help you accept change and therefore, not suffer, wallowing in disempowering thoughts of what used to be. Nature has its course. We are part of nature. Accepting what is will help you to find peace in the present moment. Ask yourself how you can be grateful for where I am right now? Life is about growing. On the outside, you may not feel that way! On the inside, where your true vibrancy and life comes from, you can cultivate inner peace. Inwardly, you can grow and flourish. That light inside of you will radiate outward to others.

A Prayer for Acceptance

Dear God,

As I take this time to be still, help me to let go of anxiousness to feel your peace.

Your Word says that you are love and where there is love there can be no fear.

Help me to let go of fear and receive your perfect love.

I come before you with heaviness because of being hurt by others.

Help me to accept the affect that their actions have had in my life and to let go of this hurt.

Holding onto past hurts—Holding onto resentments and judgments weighs me down.

I release this hurt.

I release this weight on my body and spirit. I ask your love to carry me.

I let go of hurt, resentment, and judgment.

I forgive those who have hurt me.

Because I practice awareness in all areas of my life, I am aware of self-criticism or poor choices.

I accept my actions. I forgive myself and let go of poor choices or self-criticism.

To receive or accept love, I let go of building walls of self-protection.

Help me to receive and accept love.

Help me to freely give love.

Help me not to strive for perfection but to make progress each day.

I accept the choices I make.

I can trust myself.

I make good choices.

Each day, help me to step into the glorious person you created me to be.

I accept and find comfort in knowing that I am completely loved with your divine, perfect love.

Amen

Secret 3

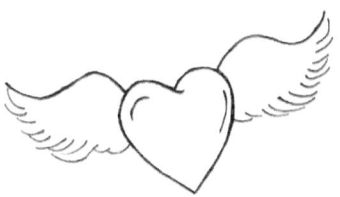

Throw Away the Scale, Let Go of Judgments

For many women (for me especially), weighing every week or (gasp) every day, can be a formula for disaster. As I mentioned before, I don't own a scale. I know that if I am eating well and exercising, I can maintain my current weight.

The scale holds huge psychological power. I stated earlier that the scale was my judge and jury. I gave power to the scale and let it affect my emotions for the entire day. The number, most of the time, would cause self-judgments. For me, it was confirmation of my unworthiness, lack of discipline, and that I was a failure. It was a measuring stick for self-worth and self-esteem.

But, you may think: how will I gauge my progress? How will I be accountable if I don't step on the scale every day or every week?

You'll know the progress you are making by feeling better, having more energy, and your clothes will become looser. From my experience, stepping on the scale every day or even every week is one of the biggest mistakes that you can make. Why? We give the scale power. Here are two scenarios.

When the Number Doesn't Change

If the number is the same, you may be okay with that or you may feel frustrated. Weight loss is not happening fast enough. This could lead to an attitude of, what's the use? Rarely do you say, "Oh, my body is just adjusting as I'm doing all the things I need to do with healthy eating and exercising each day." No! We want to be thin and we want to be thin now!

When the Number Goes Up

That reading can mean a day that is set up to be a disaster. All the self-criticism kicks into gear. Perhaps you have been eating well and exercising and you've gained weight because of simply eating something that was salty, retaining water in the form of extra weight.

If you are a woman, this stepping on the scale may be during that time of the month. It's natural to gain weight. This weight will go away after the menstrual cycle. Or maybe you had a pint of Ben & Jerry's ice cream the night before or had two glasses of wine or can't recall how much bread you had at dinner. Let the self-loathing begin. This reaction to gaining on the scale can send you in one of two directions:

1. To keep on course and realize that your weight naturally fluctuates

2. Tell yourself that you need to make better choices, today is a new day
3. Go on a binge and undo your previous efforts.

The binge may not start out as a binge. You may say that you aren't going to eat AT ALL to make up for your transgressions. This may work for breakfast and lunch, but by dinner time you will be starving and that's when the binging can happen. Not eating all day can turn into eating all night.

When the Number Goes Down

Forget about all this bad news stuff. Let's say the scale reports that you've lost a pound or two or three. You are elated. You're giving yourself a high five. You break into a victory dance and praise yourself for being conscientious and disciplined with eating well and exercising well. This reaction to losing on the scale can also send you in one of two directions:

1. To keep on course and continue to make good choices, or,
2. To celebrate with food, especially food that you have restricted and go on a binge.

After this indulgence, the weight loss from the previous day could be obliterated. And thus, the cycle continues of sabotaging your progress.

Here's what it looks like in an illustration:

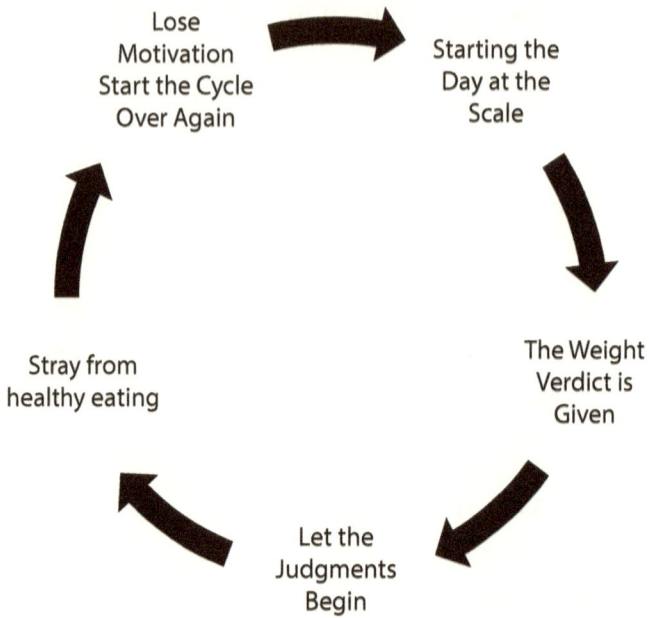

The number is the first of many judgments. Depending on that number, the judgments will be more severe. They won't be limited to weight. These judgments will be comparing yourself to others, comparing your body, your brain, your actions, your roles in life to everyone else's. The self-talk is something like, *I'll never look like* _____, *I'm a failure, I'll never lose weight, I'm an idiot, I have no self-control, how can God really love me*—insert your favorite self-loathing statements here. This initial step on the scale can be like a huge snowball collecting momentum and growing, rolling downhill. Your self-esteem also goes downhill.

If you have made the decision to lose weight, there is no magical time frame for reaching your goal. You may have five pounds or two-hundred pounds to lose. I mentioned that the thirty pounds I struggled with just melted away (over how long of a period, I don't

Secret 3 – Throw Away the Scale, Let Go of Judgments

recall because I wasn't measuring). In saying that, I stuck with listening to my body, stopping when I felt full, eating reasonable portions, exercising, and not focusing on the scale.

When you eat well and exercise, you will begin to notice the changes in your clothes. With steady, consistent progress, one day you will wake up and your clothes will be loose. One day, they may even be too big to wear. It seems like a miracle. It's almost like it happened overnight. But it didn't happen overnight. Your body had to adjust to this new routine of good nutrition and exercise. The same goes for the weight you gained in the past; only it wasn't a miracle. It was a nightmare. It seemed like you gained weight overnight, but it took time.

Taking the barrier of the scale out of the equation will take harsh judgments away. These judgments will sabotage your progress. Here's what the improved cycle looks like:

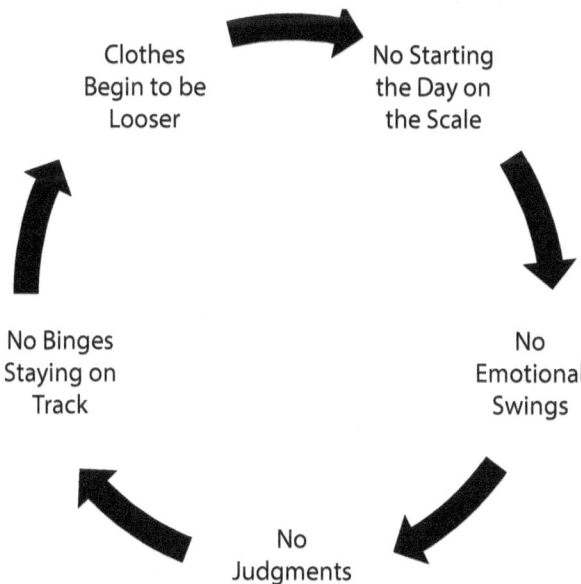

The only time I step on a scale is at my doctor's office. That's maybe once or twice a year. It's funny; I still dread the thought of getting on the scale. The scale still holds some power in that regard. I take off my shoes and jacket and make sure I'm going to be as light as possible when I step on the scale. When the number shows and it's the same as last year, there is an itty bitty part of me that wants to be surprised that I am at the same weight. For me, it's really so freeing to have left the scale behind.

All of our bodies are different. We are all unique. So, it's hard to say what that number should be. I know there are charts that physicians have for what is a healthy weight. There are also measurements such as BMI (Body Mass Index) that relate to your weight versus your height for what is considered a 'normal' weight and how that relates to mortality and diseases. Also, having abdominal fat is of great concern because of increased risk of cancers, heart disease, diabetes and liver disease. What's important is determining what the best weight is for you and being as healthy as you can be. I believe that all of us have a set point that is ideal for us. When you reach it and stay there, it can become your new set point. I have reset that set point over time.

You may be addicted to stepping on the scale. You may be afraid that if you don't have the scale, you won't know if you are making progress. (I had a woman CPA that is all about numbers. She shared with me that the scale didn't pose a problem for her. In her numbers-driven world, she needed that measurement.) You may, however, use the scale to reinforce feelings of unworthiness. The number is confirmation of your lack of self-discipline. You are locking

Secret 3 – Throw Away the Scale, Let Go of Judgments

yourself in a little box that is keeping you from freedom until you break the cycle.

About the word discipline. I've used it a couple of times here. I've also had people comment on my weight loss and say to me, "I'm just not disciplined like you are." The word brings up the meaning of sticking to rules or being punished as in being disciplined. I used to think of discipline in that way, too. But the root word comes from the Latin, discipulus which means pupil. From that word comes disciple. When we see the word disciple, it usually implies someone that followed Jesus. But a disciple is someone who follows and practices the teachings of his or her teacher or mentor. I've even heard it said that *being a disciple is following something you love.* So, being disciplined in adopting a healthy lifestyle means loving yourself. Doesn't that inspire you to be disciplined?

The 12-step recovery programs have been so effective because there are steps to practice. They also involve surrendering to a Power greater than ourselves. You are not on this journey alone. The ten secrets shared here are spiritual practices to incorporate as daily habits. The prayers at the end are to reinforce that you are not alone. You have a Higher Power in God to help you and companion you.

Let me offer a suggestion: be disciplined in treating yourself with loving kindness, and letting go of judgmental thoughts. **Think less about your weight and that goal number and focus on living your life.** Eat good, nutritious food. Find exercise that you can enjoy. Let go of the scale and its power over you.

The truth is that our weight fluctuates each day. Salt can cause a water-weight gain. Depending on where we are in our menstrual cycle, menopausal, post, pre, whatever; there are going to be certain times of the month that we gain considerable weight, not to mention that we may feel like a beached whale (that was my analogy).

I had felt that way many times before a workout, complaining to Rik about how fat I was. He would just shake his head and tell me that I certainly did not look like a beached whale and that I would feel better next week. Sure enough, I'd be bouncing into his gym the next week feeling good and he would just laugh. Old habits are hard to die, especially when hormones are talking!

Rik would say to me, "You look lean today." I'd say, "Oh, it's this shirt. The angles make me look lean." He'd reply, "Why do you women do that???" I caught myself and changed my response. "Thank you." I'd say in return.

Rik had a lot of female clients. He shared that, without exception, every woman has a different perception of herself compared to reality, especially around that time of the month. Almost every woman feels awful. Since I walked in the door, Rik had never asked me to step on the scale.

When you begin to trust yourself and keep plugging away, you will begin to feel a difference in your clothes. When you let go of judgments, from the scale and from your own self-talk, your body, mind, and soul will also become lighter. This is the journey to true freedom.

What you are adopting is a lifestyle that will last a lifetime. Focus every day (sometimes every moment) on making progress. If a day goes by and you slip, you won't focus on slipping. Instead, you focus on all the good things you are doing and how you are taking care of yourself.

They used to say that it takes twenty-one days to make a change or form a habit. But science has shown that it takes more like sixty-six days to form a new habit. As you take small steps every day, your new behaviors will become a habit. When you free your mind from the judgment of the scale, losing weight becomes less of a struggle.

Letting Go of the Perfection Bug

Have you been bitten by the perfection bug? We've talked about the marketing world's image of perfection. Added to this is an imaginary perfect bar that we hold in our minds.

I am a recovering perfectionist. I have no idea when I was bitten by the perfection bug. Maybe it goes back to third grade when I had a couple of C's on my report card and my father wrote a note to my teacher that said, "I am confident that Jackie has more within her and will do better. I will make sure that she does."

Perfectionism is an ugly habit. Striving to be perfect opens us up to an all or nothing attitude. I know I used to think if I can't be perfect then I won't do it, whatever "it" was.

If we allow perfection to rule our lives, we will miss opportunities. Instead of thinking we are not good enough, we need to adopt a new mantra, that we *are* good enough. *We are enough.*

In the mind, our perfection bar sabotages our weight loss efforts and self-esteem. "I ate bread and butter before dinner. I blew it. I wasn't perfect." Let the binging begin.

Or, "I messed up at work. I lost it and screamed at my kids." Let all the judgments fly: "You're a failure. You're a lousy mother."

This dialogue of imperfection fosters in the mind. That is why it is so important to get out of your mind and into your spirit. There is a verse from Matthew 5:48 that says, "Be perfect, therefore, as your heavenly Father is perfect."

But, Jackie, you just said to not dwell on being perfect and now I'm supposed to be perfect as in God perfect??? In this case, the word perfect comes from a Greek word meaning to fully ripen or mature.

Like beautifully ripe apples, consider the fruits of the Spirit: love, joy, peace, patience, kindness, generosity, faithfulness, gentleness, and self-control. Listening to your spirit will bypass the negative mind that tells you that you don't measure up. You'll respond to the critical judgments with a "mature" response and not a critical reaction.

Instead of judging the act of eating too much bread and butter, you can lovingly say, "I'll savor every bite of my dinner and stop when I'm full. I'll take home what I don't finish." Or, "I won't have dessert now." Or, "Bread is too tempting, I'll ask them not to put it on the table next time."

If you yell at your children or messed up at work, make it right as quickly as possible. That's what a "perfect," mature person would do. These are spiritual responses because they come from the Spirit of love, gentleness, and self-control.

I'd re-connected with my best friend from kindergarten through high school and another friend from grade school because of a high school reunion. During a dinner conversation, I mentioned that I wished I could have the last 10 years to do over again. We all agreed that we didn't want to go back to high school, or our 20s, or 30s.

I asked them what was the biggest thing they've learned in the last 40 years. Tracey said, "Not to sweat the small stuff." Marsha said, "Material things don't matter, relationships do." I said, "I wish I hadn't held onto being perfect and lived more in the present moment instead of worrying about the future. I wished I had not tried so hard to make things happen, but that I would have allowed things to

Secret 3 – Throw Away the Scale, Let Go of Judgments

happen." Added to that would have been not wasting so much time and energy worrying about my weight and appearance.

I would call that a mature conversation. That's because we had *ripened* over the years. Summed up in one word—perfect. In this case, may you be bitten by a *new perfection bug*.

Remember the first secret of awareness. Be aware of how you talk to yourself. Be aware of what you are eating. Follow up with the second secret of acceptance. Accept that you have been judgmental and strive to stop the judgments. You'll find the process will become easier in not only stopping judgments that you make about yourself, but how you make general judgments and judge other people.

Let go of the scale and instead, surrender to a Higher Power. Ask God's help to release you from judgments. If you continue to struggle with a judgmental view of God, it's not easy to surrender! I let go of that image as I spend time with God through my morning writing and meditation. Out of that time came a book called *God Notes – Daily Doses of Divine Encouragement*. There is a word each day written as a love note from God. The word Judge was appropriate for this chapter.

Judge

People will judge you by your religion or beliefs.
They will judge you by your appearance.
They will judge you by your speech.
They will judge you by your actions.
Even worse, you will judge your every action;
Judge your own decisions,
Judge your appearance,
And judge your abilities.
You may think that I judge your every move.
I am not the great judge.
You, on the other hand, have become quite an expert!
Stop being a judge.
You are precious, one-of-a-kind, whole, beautiful, and powerful beyond measure.
If I had a verdict, that is My final one.

Quieting the mind will help in overcoming negative self-talk and judgments. We'll talk about that in the next chapter.

The following cartoon is a reminder to stop judging.

Secret 3 – Throw Away the Scale, Let Go of Judgments

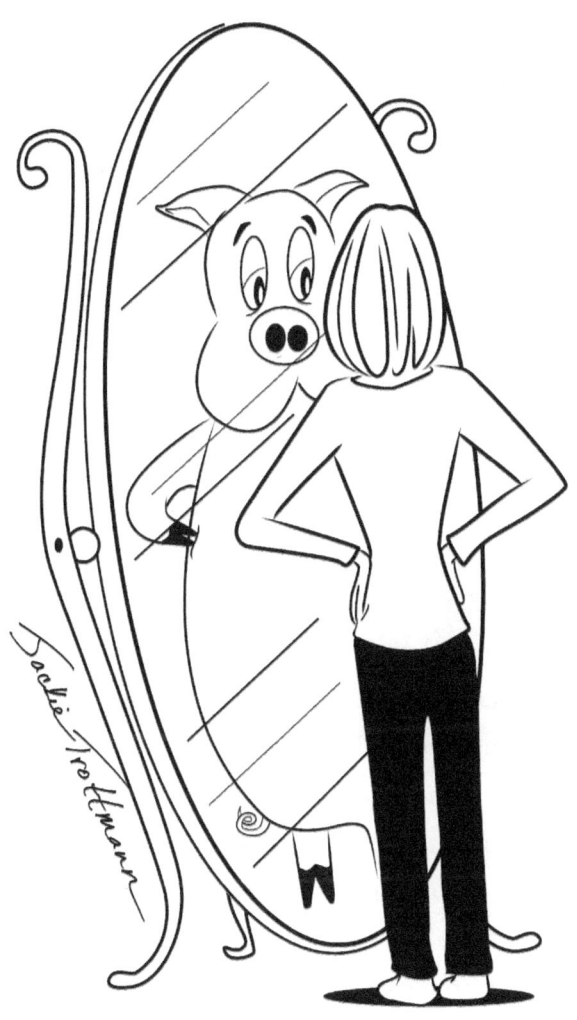

What did you say honey?
I do <u>not</u> have a poor self image!

Prayer to Let Go of Judgments

Dear God,

Help me to truly understand that there is no one else like me.

Because no one else is like me, help me to not compare myself to others.

When I compare myself to others, I'm passing judgment that is not true.

I rob myself of joy.

I release comparing myself to others so that I can become all that you created me to be.

If I judge every action I take, judge or criticize others, or believe that *you* are judging my every action, I am not able to be free.

I let go of judgments.

As I let go of judgments, I receive love.

As I let go of judgments, I receive peace.

As I let go of judgments, I receive joy.

As I let go of judgments, I receive patience.

As I let go of judgments, I receive kindness.

As I let go of judgments, I receive self-control.

Each moment, help me to continue to make better choices.

As I listen to the still, small voice inside of me, I receive guidance.

As I practice awareness each day, I become aware of the judgments that I hold onto.

As I practice acceptance, I'm able to accept that I have been judgmental or held onto judgments.

Now I can let them go.

Loving God, I release my judgments so that I can receive your peace and guidance and become *truly* free.

Amen

Secret 4

Learn to Be Still, Let Go, and Trust by Practicing Meditation

Until we learn to be still, we may never confront the issues that are simmering below the surface of our psyches. Our senses are constantly bombarded, and we lack quiet time. Yet, it is in the quiet and the stillness that we gain strength. It is in the stillness that we can commune with our Creator. "Be still and know that I am God." (Psalm 46:10)

In Hebrew *be still* means to let go or surrender. We can find comfort in knowing that God is in charge. But there is another mention of *be still* used in Mark 4:39. This time, the phrase is used by Jesus. I found this definition quite shocking and funny at the same time.

Our pastor's sermon focused on this passage. The story starts with Jesus healing many people and speaking to the crowds. He requested that he and the disciples take a boat across the water. On the journey Jesus fell asleep. A great storm came up and the disciples were afraid that they would perish. They woke up Jesus and he immediately rebuked the wind and said to the sea, "Peace! Be still!" The wind ceased and there was a dead calm.

Our pastor explained that in the Greek translation *be still* meant hush or in modern slang, *shut up!* But it makes perfect sense. How many times do we have thoughts that won't shut up? *I'll never lose weight. I can't believe I'm dieting again. Nobody loves me. I'm too old. I'm too young,* are examples of just some of the endless chatter. Be still!

In order to be still, you must set aside time each day to be quiet and still. Time is a precious resource and everyone seems to be time poor. Our lives are filled with many responsibilities and commitments. Being still may seem like doing nothing. That's how I used to view it until I found the power that comes from spending time being still in God's presence. God speaks to us in the stillness. Our souls are renewed in silence.

Because my home environment was out of my control growing up, I tried to control everything else in my power. *Surrendering* or *letting go* were not words in my vocabulary.

Prior to practicing meditation, I used to be a huge multi-tasker. My attention was rarely focused on one task. For instance, I used to try to send an email and listen to a conference call at the same time. My attention was divided. The goal was to be more efficient, but the result was being ineffective. I was always go, go, go and do, do, do. There was no time to just be.

Meditation can help quiet or shut up the mind. Meditation is a powerful tool for weight loss; it's an even more powerful tool for life. We have upwards of 60,000 thoughts a day. That's just our thoughts. Through the advancement of technology, media's intrusiveness can be compared to an assault. We are exposed to between 2,500 and

5,000 advertising messages each day. Those numbers increase daily. It's no wonder that we have lost our ability to think for ourselves.

While traditional prayer is a very important part of a spiritual life, listening is even more important. In traditional prayer we are doing all the talking; in meditation, we can hear God speaking to us. *I like to say that prayer is talking to God. Meditation is listening to God.*

Through meditation, we can also practice breathing. We can't survive without oxygen. While our hearts work at pumping blood throughout our bloodstream, oxygen cleanses our lymph system, which carries oxygen to all of our cells. Oxygen helps cells release toxins in our bodies through our lymph filter system.

Have you ever wondered about the expression, *a cleansing breath*? True, deep, abdominal breathing is a cleansing process.

Meditation reduces stress, anxiety, and depression. Just like the cleansing breath, meditation cleanses the mind from cluttered thoughts. Listening and being quiet brings clarity. In the beginning, it's also not easy. The reason why it is called practicing meditation is because it takes practice!

Our world is very fast-paced, busy, and noisy. Getting quiet takes an adjustment. But for those practicing meditation and learning to be still like I do on a regular basis, they would testify that it becomes an indispensable priority in their lives. Our bodies and entire life can be transformed through the practice of meditation.

Some immediate benefits to quieting the mind are: listening to your body (in the form of being hungry, thirsty, tired, etc.), becoming less reactive to situations, feeling greater peace, becoming less judgmental, feeling more love and compassion, feeling less stress and less anxious. Stated simply, learning to be still can help us recognize God's Spirit and the fruits of the Spirit which are: love, joy, peace, patience, kindness, generosity, faithfulness, gentleness, and self-control.

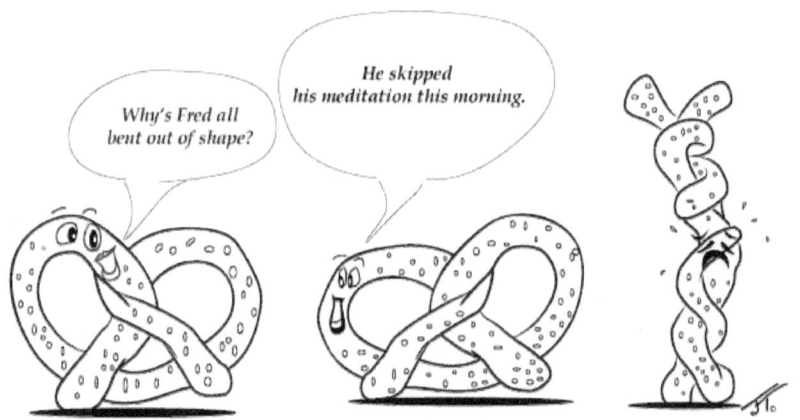

Since silencing the negative, anxious and obsessive thoughts is not always an easy process, I've developed three recorded, guided meditation CD (or download) options to help quiet the mind. All are specifically designed to experience a deeper relationship with God. The first, Be Still, is based on the Bible verse, Psalm 46:10, "Be Still and Know that I am God."

The second recorded, guided meditation CD (or download) is in the form of affirmation prayers. (You may have purchased it with this book.) It is called *Let it Go, 10 Meditative Affirmations to Let Go and Let God*. These affirmations will help to reprogram the mind, to let go of the past and behaviors that don't serve you and embrace behaviors to empower you. (These are the prayers at the end of each chapter.)

The third is in a guided prayer as well as a guided time of silence or contemplation. This is called Trust. These meditations will help you to relax and trust God, trust yourself, and trust others. Listen to samples and purchase at JackieTrottmann.com

Quieting the mind will remove the obsessive thoughts about food, weight, and appearance. All these unhealthy, cluttered thoughts can be cleared away.

Earlier I stated that recovery was surrendering. In order to overcome our addictions and problems, we need help from a Power much greater than our selves. Surrender doesn't mean quitting or even giving up control. *Surrendering means letting go of the struggle.* "My yoke is easy and my burden is light." (Matthew 11:30). A yoke was used to bind two oxen together. This bind joined the labor into one combined, powerful effort.

Too often, we lose sight of our connection to God. We can think of God being up there or out there instead of realizing God's love and power is within us. God's Spirit is one with us. God delights in us surrendering to him. He wants nothing more than to have a relationship with us and to show us what true power means. Through God we can overcome all obstacles. We don't have to make it through our life's journey on our own. We don't have to feel overwhelmed and alone.

If you grew up with an image of God like I had, it's understandable how you can turn away. Let me offer these verses of encouragement to reintroduce you to the God that I know.

Jeremiah 29:11 says, "For surely I know the plans I have for you, says the Lord, plans for your welfare and not for harm, to give you a future with hope."

These are some of my favorite verses describing God's true nature from 1 John 4:16-18: "God is love, and those who abide in love abide in God, and God abides in them. There is no fear in love, but perfect love casts out fear; for fear has to do with punishment, and whoever fears has not reached perfection in love. We love because he first loved us."

The emptiness and void that we hunger and thirst (literally) for can never be met through another person, job or material possessions. It's a spiritual hunger that only our Creator can fill. The Psalmist writes: "As a deer longs for flowing streams, so my soul longs for you, O God." Psalm 41:1. And Matthew 5:6 says, "Blessed are those who hunger and thirst after righteousness, for they will be filled."

When you learn to be still, when you learn to let go and trust, you can trust yourself and your good choices. You can trust a God who loves you and wants only the best for you. When you spend time in God's presence, your soul is filled. The impulses to reach for a drink, to over-eat, to continue obsessive thoughts and addictive behaviors are gone. You can lay your burdens at the feet of your Creator. When you do, your mind, body and spirit are lighter. You will discover the inner peace that the apostle Paul describes in Philippians 4:7, "And the peace of God, which surpasses all understanding will guard your hearts and your minds."

A Prayer to Let Go

Dear God,

In this moment, I let go of all thoughts and concerns.

When I let go, I am able to receive.

When my hands are formed into tight fists, I cannot open my hands to receive anything.

When I hang onto tight control,

When I close off my heart and my spirit,

I cannot receive your blessings for me.

I let go to receive your blessings.

Letting go in this moment, I receive your loving presence around me and within me.

Help me to let go when I am feeling overwhelmed, so that I may receive your peace.

Help me to let go when I feel fear so that in fear's place I may receive love and courage.

I let go of problems and challenges in order to receive your guidance and clarity.

I let go and trust you.

I will not fall.

You will catch me.

I let go and trust in the still, small voice inside of me.

Help me not to struggle but to surrender my struggle to you.

I gladly receive this gift of letting go and letting you lead me and guide me.

Amen

Secret 5

Use Moderation, Listen to Your Body, Eat What You Crave

The generations born prior to the 1920's and 1930's exemplified great examples of moderation and delayed gratification. Today, many people are experiencing large amounts of debt because of living beyond their means. These generations purchased something only when they had the money, with actual cash.

Perhaps it was because many lived through the Great Depression. Their moderation mindset also included eating in moderation. The food they ate didn't come out of a package. It was real food. A daily bacon and egg breakfast was prepared in moderation, compared to the large-portion-size meals offered in restaurants today.

It's important to be sure to eat a breakfast, lunch, and dinner which are moderate in size and include a full array of fresh vegetables, protein, complex carbohydrates, fruit, fats (particularly healthy fats like avocados, olive oil, other nuts and seeds) and some dairy; barring no food allergies or other issues. Depending on your metabolism, some people may be better served eating more frequently, spreading out meals throughout the day.

Food is the body's fuel. If you let your car run out of gas, it won't go anywhere. If you don't feed your body with enough fuel in the form of good nutrition, you won't function at the highest level possible.

For me, I find it helpful to eat my dinner before seven o'clock each night. The benefits are that this gives the body's digestive system time to do its work, burning more calories instead of slowing down to go into sleep mode. Also, going to bed and lying down too quickly after a sizable meal increases the chance for stomach acid to travel up the esophagus causing heartburn or gastro esophageal reflux disease. Of course, when that happens, that means sleep is interrupted.

Hydrating the body is equally important. Many times we feel hungry when we are in fact thirsty. Sometimes a glass of water is what our body needs.

Learning to be still and practicing meditation helps to get in tune with the body. I mentioned that until I discovered yoga, I had never listened to my body or felt hunger. I had short-circuited the body's natural mechanism that tells us when we're hungry and when we've had enough to eat. God gave us an amazing body that regulates our food intake just like in other animals. When's the last time you saw a fat bunny, deer, or fox?

If you do have a craving, eat what you crave. The key is to savor and enjoy it. In the beginning of this process, don't keep problem food in the house.

Secret 5 – Use Moderation, Listen to Your Body, Eat What You Crave

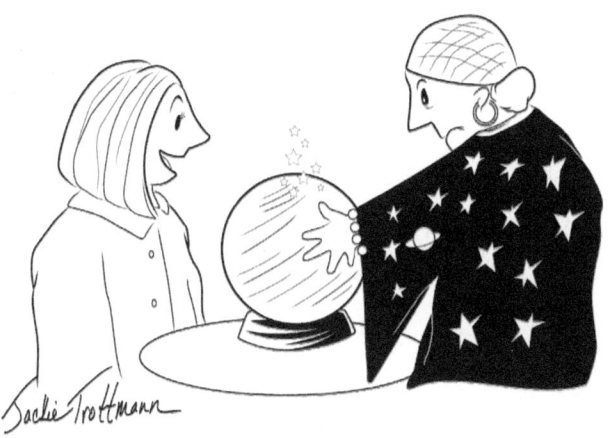

*If it says I'm gaining all of my weight back,
then I'm headed right for a double fudge sundae when we're done.*

In the past, when I was going to embark on yet another diet program that was going to get me to the magic goal weight that I rarely reached on the scale (but always reached on my driver's license), I would go on a binge. I inhaled every possible food that would be restricted from a "diet" as if I would never be able to eat it again. In the process, I would gain an additional five pounds before I started. Sounds like pretty crazy thinking, until you understand how the mind works.

What happens when you're told you can't have something? You immediately have to have it! You may recall a rather well-known story from the second chapter of Genesis where the first man and woman were told not to eat fruit from a certain tree. A few verses later, what did they do? They ate from the tree. We all know how that turned out!

Restrictive diets, more often than not, lead to failure. Restrictive calorie intake and restrictive foods can lead to gaining the lost weight back. If you reincorporate all the foods and quantities that made you gain weight in the first place, the weight is bound to come back. Losing weight needs to involve embracing a healthy lifestyle change to nourish the body.

Getting back to the craving subject, let's say you have a craving for Oreo cookies. Don't buy the tsunami-size bag of Oreos. If you do have a craving, however, buy the snack-size found at most convenience stores, drug stores or supermarket checkout isles.

Eat one Oreo very slowly. If you want, eat two, but stop there. Take your time to savor the cookie. Then tell yourself, "I really enjoyed that! I don't need to eat any more, because I know what an Oreo tastes like. It has satisfied my craving. The second Oreo, third Oreo or twenty-third Oreo tastes the same!" Then throw the rest of the cookies away. If you feel confident that you can take the remainder of the package home without eating them immediately, then go right ahead. But, if you know that the opened package of cookies will become too much of a temptation, then it's best to throw them away.

Earlier I shared how I resisted eating a piece of pie when that's what I was craving. The result was taking in a lot more calories and ultimately eating the pie anyway. So, if you have a craving, satisfy it. If that craving leads to eating an entire bag or box of something, your craving is not about food. There is an affirmation prayer at the end of this chapter to turn to when you have insatiable cravings.

Once you've made the switch from a diet filled with lots of processed foods, sugars, artificial sweeteners, and fat-laden fast-food, you'll find that the cravings for unhealthy food will diminish. Your body will crave nourishment and you will want to fuel your body with healthier choices for the simple fact that healthier choices make you feel better. *The freedom to eat* means having the freedom to eat what you want without guilt, self-loathing, or gaining back the lost weight. That is the result of making good choices for your ultimate health and well-being.

Work on changing your mindset about the act of wasting food, if that is an issue for you. If you eat more than you should, it will do more harm to your health. I am not proposing that you need be wasteful. The reality, unfortunately, is that portion sizes in the United States are huge. Consider cutting portions in half and putting it in a to-go container, **before** you begin to eat your meal. Better yet, split portions with a friend or family member. You'll save money, too.

I have mentioned that I participated in many diet programs, some with pre-packaged foods and some without. My intent is not to discourage anyone from joining one of the weight loss programs available. If that is something that you want to do, by all means do it, if you believe it will help you to get on track. Ultimately, you are the only person who holds the power to make good choices when it comes to your health and well-being. Until you look at food as a wondrously, pleasurable means to obtain sustenance for each day, you will continue to abuse food and play the endless gaining and losing game. All the programs I joined worked for me in taking off the weight. Unfortunately, my behavior did not change, and I was not able to keep the weight off.

A Prayer for Letting Go of Cravings

Dear God,
Thank you for my amazing body.
When I take time to be still—I can hear my breathing.
I can feel my heart beating.
I am grateful for my legs, which take me where I need to go.
I am grateful for my hands which help me accomplish so many tasks.
I am grateful for my wonderful mind.
I am grateful for my heart that physically sustains my life.
I am grateful for my heart that speaks the truth as I listen.
My body holds my soul. That's why I want to care for my body.
Thank you for the miracle that my body tells me what it needs as I listen.
When I pay attention, I am aware of my body's signals.
Thank you for the variety of foods that provide pleasure and sustenance for my body.
Help me to move my body every day and give my body the exercise it needs.
Help me to practice moderation in eating, drinking, and exercise.
Help me to know the difference between physical hunger and emotional hunger.
When I feel empty I ask your help to fill my hunger.
God, please fill me with your peace and loving Spirit.
Help me to let go of my obsessive or anxious thoughts.
When I let go of these thoughts, I am able to receive peace.
As I continue to listen, my body will tell me what it needs physically.
As I continue to listen, my spirit will tell me what I need emotionally.

Thank you, loving God, for supplying my every need.
Amen

Now that you have become aware of behaviors, accepted poor choices or accepted past hurts and let them go, you're letting go of judgments, not allowing the scale to hold you hostage, you're listening to your body, quieting your mind, and are on the road to your goal weight or are at your goal weight and want to maintain your weight, here are some big questions: *Who are you? Who is the ultimate you that has been buried under the physical, emotional and spiritual weight that you carried?*

Secret 6

Discover Who You Really Are, Discover Your Strengths and Talents

If you've ever asked, "Who am I?" does your answer appear to be something **you** created? Or is it something created by the family, the environment, media, social circles, or other areas of influence in your life?

From my perspective, I believe many people are lost, meaning not living as the person they are meant to be. Our culture tries to influence our view and shape our thoughts into the 'ideal' person, using the power of the media. I found this to be true for myself as I shared my constant comparison to images in magazines.

Around the time of my birth was the birth of television into consumers' homes. The influence of media had such a profound effect on my self-esteem, even with only a handful of television networks and magazines. With the explosion of twenty-four-hour media sources and the continuing rapid advancement of technology, social media has also been added to the mix of mediums that can't help but influence our behavior in not only how we see ourselves, but how we think others see us.

I recall an Oprah interview with an author where they discussed being your authentic self. That was the first time that I heard those words. I thought, *what a bunch of psychobabble*. Obviously, I was not in the right place mentally or emotionally to receive the message. Today, being authentic means everything to me.

To be honest, I didn't jump on the social media bandwagon. I had done so much internal work in excavating my buried self-esteem that getting people to "like me" seemed absurd. I truly understand the huge benefits of social media; to get in touch with distant friends and family, to expand one's sphere of influence and marketing reach, but I hope that you can appreciate the initial irony for me.

What concerns me most about social media is an issue that was validated by my son. We were talking at dinner and I was asking him about social media, since his phone seems to be an extension of his thumbs. He very casually explained, as if everyone knew this, that people have two personas, one when they are in front of people and one they project in social media. That's what I was afraid he was going to say. That, of course, is a survey of one. But research is showing that social media can cause depression because of peer pressure and even envy in comparing one's life and accomplishments to others.

Social media is also another form of marketing. Having worked in sales and marketing for over three decades, the role of marketing is to influence behavior and motivate consumers to purchase a product or service. In the United States, we are particularly driven by consumerism. We have become a society that believes the latest and greatest thing will make us happy. What car we drive, the clothes we

Secret 6 – Discover Who You Really Are, Discover Your Strengths and Talents

wear, what zip code we live in, the *brands* we consume, all outwardly define us.

At the same time, many people are very much in debt. Are people happier with all their your material things? This includes our weight as well. How many times have you attempted to lose weight because of an upcoming wedding, vacation, reunion or other event? You might have even been successful. After the event was over, however, did you maintain the weight loss?

Oftentimes, people lose weight, but haven't yet discovered who they are. Many change their outward appearance, but haven't tuned into their true essence. Losing weight is supposed to be the answer to happiness. I believe this is the core reason why so many people regain their weight very soon afterwards. I know that's why I was unable to keep the weight off. I had changed on the outside but not on the inside. Losing weight was purely to look good. I thought it was my answer to happiness.

For me, the weight was a symptom of a deeper weight that I carried. My preoccupation with weight loss was blocking the true issues I needed to deal with on the inside. It was a distraction. I had no self-awareness of an interior life. The seduction of outward beauty and success was all-consuming.

What's important to grasp is that the real person, the real you and I are not the body we live in. Once we realize that, we are free from being so concerned with our outward appearance. Our primary purpose for being is to find out who we are and step into our ultimate potential. That means using all of your strengths and talents to bring love and joy to this world. Yes, the world needs you!

You may be thinking, *strengths? I don't have any strengths.* Have you taken the time to explore this thought? Overall, in our society, we tend to focus on weaknesses in order for us to improve. The problem with that thinking is that most weaknesses don't necessarily get stronger.

I would venture to guess that almost everyone has had this experience, when they received a report card in school. On the card were four A's and one B or four B's and one C. What did your parents focus on? The B or C. A few seconds of praise (maybe) were given to the top grades, then the lecture started on improving the weakness.

On a personal level, math was never an area of strength for me. Put an Excel spreadsheet in front of me and my eyes will glaze over. As a business major and now a business owner, math is an extremely important part of running a successful business. I've taken classes to try to improve, but this area is not a strength for me. Rather than try to master, in this case, accounting, I accept this and hire people that have strengths in this area to help me. This allows me to focus on my strengths and activities that I enjoy.

Throughout my career in the corporate world, I was fortunate to participate in some great workshops and training seminars. These opportunities helped me grow and excel in the business environment, but more importantly, they helped me to have a better understanding of who I am.

One workshop that had a profound effect was when I was working at Clear Channel Radio. It was completely focused on strengths. Weaknesses were mentioned only to say that focusing on a weakness will never make one stronger. The report card scenario I mentioned earlier had always bugged me. It raised the question of, "Why can't I be good at everything?" Or worse, "What's wrong with me?"

Through the workshop, I discovered how I am wired. It helped me to understand why I act and perform the way I do. Each strength and its definition resonated with me. This was enlightening to me because it answered that *why* I couldn't be good at everything, and the most important question, "What is wrong with me?" The answer was that there was nothing wrong with me! I'm wired a certain way. We all have our own DNA. This was liberating!

Since the training was taken by the entire management team, I also had a better understanding of how everyone else was wired. Prior to the workshop, I had been butting heads with another sales manager. There was always some form of confrontation between us. My constant thoughts concerning him were, *why can't he be more like me? Why can't he see what I am trying to do?*

After the workshop, each manager was given a copy of all the managers' strengths. It turned out that the manager with whom I had all the conflicts was wired completely different from me. That explained why we were butting heads all the time. Once that understanding was reached, our confrontations turned to collaboration. It was amazing.

While the workshop helped me from a broad-based perspective, it was presented in the context of work and career. When I left the radio business, I started earnestly seeking deeper meaning on a psychological and spiritual level on how I was wired. There are many wonderful books and tools available to help us discover who we are. Some that have inspired me are listed in a reference section at the back of this book.

The Bible says, "Seek and you will find." Prior to seeking and finding more meaning and authenticity in my life, I had many books on success. Success was defined in the material sense of money, stature, and acquiring possessions. These books were donated to the public library as I cleared the clutter and old beliefs that did not serve me any longer. As my perspective changed, I found that most of these books did not address success from the aspect of wholeness. I believe that we are made up of a body, mind, and spirit. I let go of the books that left the spirit part out, which is the true essence of who we really are.

My new definition of success is having the peace of God, being of service to others, loving fully, and being loved in return. This includes using my talents and being creative, because God is the ultimate Creator. It is putting my complete trust in God to lead me and guide me in my life to become the ultimate person God created me to be. My sincere wish is that you will find the real person within so that you may truly love and enjoy life's journey. If you are still struggling with loving yourself and accepting God's love to the fullest, I ask you to do the following. Write yourself a love letter from God.

My pastor suggested that I do this. This was an exercise that church staff members performed at a retreat. The rules were that you couldn't say anything negative. This had to be a true love letter from God. In the letter, thank God for all of your gifts and talents. See yourself as God sees you.

I have to say that it was one of the most cathartic things I have ever done. I wrote the letter in one of my journals. If I am having a particularly bad day, I will turn to the letter. Taking all the judgment away and realizing how God sees me was very profound. I urge you to write the letter.

Years after doing this exercise, I attended a month-long prayer retreat. We were told to pray for twenty minutes each day and allow God to show up. On the first day, as I settled down to pray, I asked God to give me a word. God answered. God said, "Believe." There

Secret 6 – Discover Who You Really Are, Discover Your Strengths and Talents

must have been fifty sentences that tumbled out. I was able to capture the following. I thought it might be helpful as you write your letter:

Believe you are loved.
Believe you are worthy.
Believe you are able.
Believe it's your time.
Believe I am yours.
Believe you are mine.
I believe in YOU.

This word turned into the book: *God Notes – Daily Doses of Divine Encouragement*. So, you never know where your time spent being still will lead.

When you live your life embracing who you are (and Whose you are), and using your strengths and talents, something wonderful happens. It's like being swept along in a current of spiritual flow. The struggle is gone, the anxiety is gone, the self-criticisms are gone, the emptiness is gone. You suddenly find direction and peace.

If you've taken the time to be still and stop running, if you are practicing awareness, acceptance, letting go of judgments, and paying attention to the still, small voice inside of you, you will be led and guided to the ultimate you.

If you are still feeling lost (and we all feel lost from time to time), listen even more closely to what your gut, heart, or spirit is telling you. I've found many times that it's what I *don't* want that helps me to find what I *do* want.

If participating in certain activities make you feel anxious or shut down in some way, stop participating in those activities. If, however, something makes you feel empowered and joyful, then pay attention and participate in those activities. It's really quite simple when you pay attention and bring your awareness into the present moment. (Don't forget to check the resource section at the back of the book for tools to help you discover your strengths and understand how you are wired.)

A Prayer to Discover and Use Strengths and Talents

Dear God,
I come to this place in stillness—to be in your presence.
I feel your presence all around me and within me.
Thank you for the strengths and talents you've given me.
Help me to discover and use my strengths and talents for your purpose.
When I use my strengths and talents, I feel expansive.
I feel peace.
I feel purpose.
My spirit soars.
As I focus on my strengths, I gain clarity and direction.
Help me to nurture and use my strengths and talents.
My strengths and talents are gifts from you.
My heart is filled with gratitude, and I thank you.
I ask for the opportunity to use these gifts every day and that by doing so;
I may be a blessing to others.
Amen

Secret 7

Start Loving Life

When you decide you are in love with your life, the world extends its arms wide open. People and opportunities come into your life, more than you could have ever imagined or wished. You march to your own beat, and the beat is now a beautiful melody. The discord has turned into harmony. Your mind is not filled with the clutter of judgmental thoughts, obsessing about your weight and appearance. Such a life awaits you. The choice is yours.

So, let me ask you a question.

What would you do if you weren't struggling with your weight? Do it!

Are you letting your weight stop you from doing something that you want to do?

Do you know what you want to do?

Dance?

Sing?

Paint?

Ride a horse?
Go to the pool?
Enter a cooking contest?
Go to a Broadway play?
Go on a trip to Europe?
Go on a trip across the United States?
Play golf?
Play tennis?
Write a book?

Take a few minutes to journal and explore the following topics:

1. Make a list of ten dreams or desires that you have. It could be as simple as to visit an antique store or as elaborate as climbing Mount Everest! If you feel really creative, write 100!
2. For each one, think about why you are not engaged in these activities right now.

Maybe the answer is just doing it. If you find it hard to answer, here are some questions for you to explore:

What are you afraid of?
What are you ashamed of?
Are you waiting for permission—if so, from whom?
Does it matter what people think? Why?

Review the list then create a plan to start doing each one of them. Take an action step now; such as calling to enroll in a class.

The most important thing is to live in the moment. Release your ties to the past. If you tried something and failed, let it go. If someone told you that you can't—is that really true? While it's important to learn from the past, don't be limited by the past.

"This one thing I do, forgetting those things which are behind and reaching forth unto those things which are before." Saint Paul

Many times we will say that we will do something tomorrow; or we want to make lots of plans for the future, as if the future is always brighter than the present moment. We miss out on living. So, don't focus on tomorrow.

Jesus said, "Do not worry about tomorrow, for tomorrow will worry about itself. Each day has enough trouble of its own."

We've all heard the inspirational prompt to live each day as if it is your last. Life's demands distract us from heeding this advice. It's only when we lose our health or a loved one that this invitation to live for today gets our attention.

I still attend the same gym. You may or may not have noticed that I talk about Rik in the past tense. On a Thursday, my usual workout day, I went in to work out with Rik. He seemed kind of distracted that day. When I asked him about it, he said he was thinking about re-arranging the equipment. Rik was always painting the place or moving things around, so I didn't think much of it. At the end of our routine, he stretched me out like he always did. For some reason, I held onto the feeling of his strong arms around my neck and shoulders.

The next day I had not been online at all. I received a text from my friend Steve late in the afternoon. He asked if I had heard the sad news? I texted back, no. His response was: oh my, I'm calling you. The phone rang, and Steve told me that Rik had died. It was either an aneurysm or a heart attack. He was only fifty-two years old. There was no warning. Thursday I was with him. Friday he was gone.

So, that living as if every day is your last took on much greater meaning for me. What I was most grateful for was that a few months prior was Thanksgiving. I had given Rik a card and expressed my gratitude for all he had done for me. When he died, just two months later, I was so thankful that he had known how much he meant to me.

When you experience a loss such as this, it helps to put your priorities in order. Rik used his gifts and talents to the fullest. He was a wonderful personal trainer and a wonderful human being.

Live in the present moment and make the most of it. The Psalmist says, "This is the day that the Lord has made; let us rejoice and be glad in it."

Your life is waiting to be lived. If you are waiting for permission, let me be the one to grant it to you. You have permission to pursue your dreams!

A Prayer to Start Loving Life

Dear God,
In this quiet and stillness,
I let go of the demands on my time.
I let go of anxious or cluttered thoughts.
I come to this moment with a heart filled with gratitude for my life.
Thank you, God, for creating me.
I freely receive your love and I give love.
I am filled with your peace and your presence.
Help me to focus on what is most important in my life.
When I am still, I am attentive to guidance and direction.
As I continue to open my heart and my mind,
I open myself to greater possibilities.
I appreciate the gift of life.
I appreciate all of creation.
God, fill me with your life force, power, and presence.
Help me to radiate that presence to all I come in contact with each day.
I receive this gift of life and use this gift to its fullest each day.
Amen

Secret 8

Invest in Yourself

Knowing who you are and loving your life is presented inwardly through your thoughts and feelings. You listen to the still, small voice inside of you that leads you and guides you. It is a strong and confident voice that knows the truth. You are no longer condemning yourself but are nurturing yourself. Wholeness means taking care of your mind, body, and spirit. It means investing in resources and activities to help you be the best that you can be and to live life to the fullest.

Outwardly, you express how you care for yourself. Through your outward appearance, you project your true essence to the world. Caring for your appearance does not meet the requirements communicated by the media. It is an honorable, clean, and respectful appearance of who you are.

So you're not at the ideal place you want to be with your weight. Don't let that keep you from looking good and feeling good. Buy some new clothes that look great on you right now. This means, the right fit, the right colors, the right style that defines your authentic self. There are many retailers with bargain deals, so there is no need to spend a lot of money while your shape changes. Remember, change doesn't happen overnight.

This may seem a little silly to bring up, but you'll be surprised how much better you will feel if you wear underwear that provides the support needed in all areas of the body. Some stores may offer bras and panties that look great, but don't have the fit that will make you feel comfortable all day. If you find yourself tugging and pulling on your clothes all day, that certainly doesn't look good or feel good! As your guide, remember, if it makes you feel good, then go for it; otherwise, focus on buying something that gives the right support and makes you feel better. There are many pretty and practical choices available on the market.

If your hair is one of your best features, invest in a great hairstyle and cut that represents your authentic you. If wearing makeup makes you feel good, pick products that will enhance your features and skin tone. For some, this may mean natural, clean skin. Others may enjoy facials or hair coloring. What's important is to feel good and to let your inward light shine outward for the world to see. Notice I said to **let** it shine. You don't have to **make** it shine.

Don't allow negative talk! Keep reminding yourself that you are loved unconditionally. Each day you are discovering what it means to feel connected to your Creator and in this process; you are experiencing love, joy, peace, power, and wholeness.

Time is our most precious commodity. Be careful how you invest your time. Practicing the first secret of awareness will help you to be conscious of how you spend your time and how participating in activities that are not serving you will cause you to feel bad. Invest

Secret 8 – Invest in Yourself

your time in activities that will nourish and feed your mind, body, and soul and not deplete you.

Avoid tabloids, magazines or other forms of media that propose an unrealistic view of beauty. Instead, find positive lifestyle types of media to give you new ideas and enhance your new authentic style. The same goes for camping out on social media, watching certain television programs or movies. I found the more I saturated myself with images that I couldn't attain (I will never be 5'11" except in five-inch heels) and material possessions that were not practical or true priorities like yachts or thirty-room mansions (not a heart's desire or a need for); it would still make me feel less worthy. Don't allow that to happen. Change your focus from lack to abundance by feeding your mind, body, and spirit with positive books, friends, entertainment choices, and activities.

Watch less media and move your body more often. Don't look back on your life recounting how many movies and programs you watched. Life is meant to be lived!

Invest in a personal trainer or yoga instructor and incorporate proper strength training into your exercise routine. This may seem like a luxury, but it is really an investment in your health. How much money do you spend on lattes, lunches, dinners, wine, or bottled water? Better yet, find a friend or friends and share the cost. Trainers will discount services when they train multiple clients at one time. You can hold yourselves accountable, save money, and enjoy companionship, too! By trading short-lived discretionary purchases like those mentioned for 4-8 personal training sessions a month, you will be investing in long-term health and wellness benefits. Here's what working with a personal trainer or instructor can do for you:

- Hold you accountable for your goals and desires to change your body and your mindset,
- Help you build strength and muscle mass, improving your overall health and fitness, including maintaining bone mass to help avoid osteoporosis,
- Help make sure that you are using the proper technique to prevent injury,
- Give you the results you want by varying your routine. Muscles get used to routines. They need to be worked in different ways in order to become stronger,
- Sculpt your physique as you get leaner,
- Empower your confidence and watch it go through the roof,
- You'll stand taller and be less tired,
- Improve your metabolism as you gain more muscle so that you'll be able to eat more! Muscle burns more calories!

Always be learning. In the Start Loving Life chapter we touched on dreams and goals of what you wanted to do. Invest in classes and coaches to help you achieve these goals or dreams faster.

Learning anything new, especially a huge goal like learning a language, starting a business, writing a book, or losing weight, all require learning, failing and succeeding. Working with a coach or mentor can help accelerate the process because they know the pitfalls and can help you. Plus, it's comforting to have the support, especially when you find a trusted source to help you. Find resources at JackieTrottmann.com/resources.

Remember to celebrate successes. Buy something you have always wanted, choosing something other than food or drink. Take time to acknowledge that you are transforming and are no longer repeating past behaviors. At the end of each day, focus on what progress you have made. Small action steps over time add up to huge progress. Progress is not made in huge leaps. It's made in small, consistent steps. Being in action keeps you from getting stuck.

A Prayer for Investing in Yourself

Dear God,

Thank you for the gift of life.

Thank you for my amazing body.

Help me to invest time to move my body, nourish my body, and make my body stronger.

I know that my body is a sacred vessel.

My body holds my soul.

My body holds the Holy Spirit.

Help me to be mindful of how I take care of my body.

Thank you for my amazing mind.

My mind helps me to grow in knowledge.

Help me to be careful what I feed my mind.

Thank you for my amazing spirit.

As I take this time to be still, I am open to receive your love, peace, clarity, and direction.

When I invest in this time to be still, I invest in my ability to grow.

Help me to keep growing stronger.

Help me to always be learning.

Help me to be receptive to my still, small voice that leads me and guides me.

Help me to always be mindful of your love and presence with me and within me.

Amen

Secret 9

Clear Clutter from Your Life

Clutter comes in two forms, mental clutter of the mind and physical clutter. We've already discussed mental clutter, Secret 4, Meditation, Letting Go, and Trusting. When your mind is cluttered with thoughts of worry, doubt, fear, obsessing about your weight and appearance, and thousands more, there is no room to receive peace and clarity. The thoughts that don't serve you must be cleared out to allow the thoughts that do. If physical clutter is not an issue for you, congratulations! If it is, here are tips that worked for me.

If you have a lot of clutter to deal with, don't try to tackle it all at once. It's a formula for becoming overwhelmed and not even getting started. Instead, start with a small decluttering task such as the trunk of your car, your desk, or one room.

This includes closets and cabinets, too. Energy needs space to flow and that means having free space in a medicine cabinet, book shelf or closet. Just because you don't see it, doesn't mean the bad energy is not there. Remember the basement story.

Find three boxes. Designate them as:

1 – Throw Out Now

2 – Charity

3 – Not Sure.

Begin to place items into each box. Each week, toss out the Throw Out Now box and take the Charity box to a designated charity. By the end of the week, decide what to do with the Not Sure box.

When you look at the Not Sure item, ask yourself if it truly brings you joy. Here are some other questions to help you let go and to keep the decluttering process going.

- Do I use it?
- Do I need it?
- Is it beautiful?
- Does it bring me joy?
- Is it broken, damaged, inoperable?
- If I lost it in a fire, would I replace it exactly as is?
- What kind of energy do I get from it—positive or negative?
- Will it be of pleasure or use to my heirs?

This may be a long process for some. Just like losing a significant amount of weight takes time, going through a life-time of clutter will take time. Parting with memories is not easy and must be a gentle process. As you let go of photos or letters, say a prayer to honor the relationship, then move on.

Take these questions into account when purchasing new or used items. I've already commented on credit card debt and where our culture is with this problem. Shopping can make us feel good, but that good feeling in the moment can translate to trouble. Shopping can also be an obsession whether the items are purchased in a retail store, online, or at a garage sale.

Secret 9 – Clear Clutter from your Life

I would like to say that the basement remained clutter free. It didn't. But that wasn't our fault. (Remember that sentence in Secret 2 - Acceptance?)

My son moved in after attending college. He and his stuff moved into the basement.

My mother passed away and all her stuff landed in the basement.

Robert's father passed away and all his stuff landed in the basement.

Unlike the last move, this was at least an organized mess. But it was even more overwhelming because it involved going through our parents' lifetime of possessions.

My son moved out, but several boxes of his stuff were left behind. The clutter remained until Robert and I decided to build a house together. That decision forced us to move everything out.

It was an extremely hard process. Having to do this again was also very discouraging. I found myself procrastinating until I could procrastinate no more.

The prior boxes I had moved into Robert's basement after we were married had not been touched in fourteen years. It was easy to answer those eight questions (Do I use it? Do I need it?), etc. with a big, "No."

In addition to answering the eight questions to determine whether to keep something, I discovered two powerful tips to overcome my procrastination in clearing out the clutter:

1. Have a deadline.
2. Put a time to declutter on your calendar.

Deadlines force you to get something done. That's most likely why people decide to lose weight. There's a deadline looming: a wedding, graduation, trip, etc. Deadlines give you an incentive and force you to take action.

We had a deadline to sell the house and a deadline to move into the next house. Building the house took months. It wasn't until the last four weeks prior to its completion that I got serious about clearing out the clutter in the basement. Why? Because I had a deadline and I finally put decluttering time on my calendar.

We always put important dates on our calendars, don't we? There are doctor appointments, business meetings, children's events, dates and times that we block out.

Having come from the business world, my calendar was always full of important business commitments. But there are other important activities like paying bills, cleaning the house, exercising, grocery shopping, and other tasks that are part of daily living that need to be put on the calendar too.

I would discount these activities as not important. They are, in fact, necessary and important. They also take up time during our day.

Now I am trying to be mindful and put *everything* on my calendar. Otherwise, it all stays in my head. That's mental clutter that you and I don't need.

One of the great feelings of joy and accomplishment is to check off something that you have completed.

Every year I pick a word for the year. This year's word was **simplify**. At the time, I didn't know we would be moving. This event has certainly prompted simplifying our surroundings. We are letting go of a lot of stuff that will not come with us.

There is a line from the following Let Go of Clutter Prayer that says:

Secret 9 – Clear Clutter from your Life

As I clear clutter from my mind, help me to clear physical clutter from my surroundings, because my surroundings reflect the peacefulness I feel.

Clearing clutter from your life will open up space for you to receive greater peace and abundance.

My mother left behind very few keepsakes in the form of material possessions. But she left me with many personal memories that I will always treasure in my heart.

Dealing with our parents' stuff made me truly realize what is important in life. It's not the material possessions, it's the experiences and times that we spend with the people that matter in our lives. That is where the lasting treasure lies.

For those living with someone else's clutter, ask them to get involved. Don't go through their possessions. Perhaps your example will inspire them to address the clutter in *their* lives.

Look at the clutter in your life. If you continue to be stuck in any area of your life, physically, mentally, emotionally, or in your career, clearing your clutter may help you find an answer.

A Prayer to Let Go of Clutter

Dear God,

I come before you and ask to clear my mind of cluttered thoughts.

I bring all of my awareness to be in your presence.

Help me to clear out thoughts of worry or concern.

Help me to clear out thoughts of anxiousness.

Help me to clear out fearful thoughts.

When I clear cluttered thoughts,

I am able to expand my mind.

I create space to receive love, peace, clarity, and abundant thoughts.

I feel your loving presence with me and within me.

Fill me with your peace, love, and abundance.

Help me to feel expansive and open to new possibilities.

As I clear clutter from my mind, help me to clear physical clutter from my surroundings,

because my surroundings reflect the peacefulness I feel.

Help me to release clutter to feel the lightness of your Spirit.

Amen

Secret 10

Make Life not About You Anymore

When you live your life from gratitude, you can begin to count your blessings. When your thoughts are no longer about your weight, appearance, and self-condemnation, you can switch your focus to helping and serving others. There is a great world in need, just waiting for the greatest part of who you are to be of service. The world needs you and what you have to offer!

Take a moment and stop to think about what you have in this life. Even on days when you may feel miserable, you have so much to be grateful for, especially if you live in the United States of America.

You have unlimited, clean drinking water at your disposal. Supermarkets offer almost any food you can imagine, some twenty-four hours a day. You are free to worship without fear. These things can easily be taken for granted.

At the beginning of this year, I did something I never considered before. I looked deeply at myself in the mirror. For decades, this first day of January would have marked a day of self-loathing. I would have overeaten during the holidays and would have been bulging out of my clothes. That behavior is gone.

Instead, I stood in front of the mirror and acknowledged how far I had come. I congratulated myself for being in the best shape of my life. There were no more goals of losing weight and getting into shape. No more energy wasted. I had released that burden. I was truly free.

My only regret was that I had spent so many years in the state of self-centeredness and self-loathing. My goal every New Year is to be of service, which includes helping as many people, young and old, break this same vicious cycle.

I encourage you to find ways to volunteer and help others. Not only will you provide a great service to others, but the rewards in joy and personal purpose will return to you ten-fold.

Know that you were created with unique gifts and talents to serve the greater good. We were not created to make an impression but to be an expression of what is inside of us, whatever form that takes.

As I continue to practice these ten secrets with you, may you claim God's unlimited potential to become all that God created you to be.

A Prayer to Claim Unlimited Potential

Dear God,

In this time of quiet and stillness I ask to renew my strength.
With each breath, I breathe in your presence.
God, I feel your Divine Spirit around me and within me.
I thank you that I am a part of you.
I thank you that I am connected to you.
I thank you that I am connected to all of creation.
I open my mind.
I open my heart.
I am filled with your love and appreciation.
I find peace and wholeness through your loving Spirit.
God, I receive and am filled with your peace, purpose, and power.
I ask to use my strengths and talents to help others.
I ask to be a blessing to others.
God, I thank you that I am a divine and unique expression of you.
My daily prayer is to be conscious of your loving, peaceful presence.
May I reflect your presence to others.
I claim your unlimited potential to be used in me and through me.
Amen

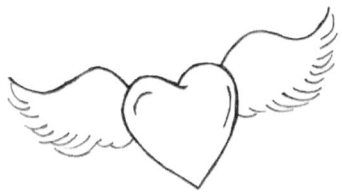

The Freedom to Eat

Imagine:
- Letting go of past hurts and pains,
- Being able to express yourself and loving it,
- Being more self-aware and aware of others,
- Understanding yourself and others better and understanding what it means to love and be loved,
- Not obsessing about how you look and what you are going to eat,
- Not stressing out about what you are going to wear because your clothes don't fit,
- Loving the holidays and going to parties,
- Feeling strong, confident and healthy,
- Looking in a mirror and liking the person you see,
- Knowing how much you are loved by God,
- Being of service to others and living your life on purpose.

If you embrace these secrets and make a little progress every day, you will move forward and begin to live a life of joy and flow.

Your life will be filled with much more than food. You will have good days and bad days. Forgive yourself and keep moving. The goal is not perfection but progress. You'll find much more than just *the freedom to eat*. I believe you will have the freedom to live the life you have always wanted or dreamed of but may have forgotten.

GOD BLESS YOU ON YOUR JOURNEY TO EXPERIENCE THE FREEDOM TO EAT!

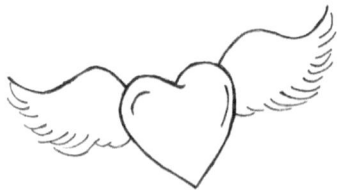

Epilogue

The *Freedom to Eat* came to fruition after I received a call from my friend, Caroline Ravelo. Our paths had crossed on several occasions. She had moved to Fort Meyers, Florida from St. Louis to follow her dreams. This involved working with authors and speakers and putting on events that focused on the mind, body, and spirit. She knew I had quit the corporate world to pursue my dream of writing, so she asked me to speak at an event she was putting on in Fort Meyers.

I was thrilled and said yes. During our conversation I told her I didn't know what to speak about. We scheduled a conference call to brainstorm some topics. As soon as I hung up the phone I knew what I wanted to talk about… *the freedom to eat*. I knew I had to share my story of how I had overcome my struggle with the physical, emotional, and spiritual weight that I carried for so long. This opportunity to speak turned into writing this book.

The conference in Fort Myers was a wonderful event filled with loving and positive energy. Many women expressed similar experiences that I share in *The Freedom to Eat*. It was rewarding to establish an instant connection and offer encouragement that there was light on the other side of their dark times.

Before leaving the hotel to return home, I picked up a magazine on Florida living. Waiting at the airport, I proceeded to look through its contents. In the first twelve pages, there were eight full-page advertisements for plastic surgeons.

When I returned from my trip, I was facing surgery to have a persistent ovarian cyst removed. I was extremely concerned whether the cyst would be benign, whether they would find anything else, and whether the surgery itself would go smoothly. Reading ads to go under a knife for the sake of fighting a losing battle to be youthful made me heartsick, because so much of our society has reached this point for a woman's self-worth.

I made it through the surgery with flying colors. Everything went as planned and the cyst was benign. The surgery was performed through a laparoscopic procedure due to my weight and size.

I share this final story because my wish for women (and men) is that we begin to take ownership of our self-worth and our health. Sure, I don't like to see lines and sags on my body that weren't there yesterday.

This is not a condemnation for anyone considering plastic surgery. If I am to honor encouraging you to make better choices and to feel good, I would admit that plastic surgery, if done well, could accomplish that. It's tempting. For me, I choose to practice the second spiritual secret of acceptance. I have the choice to accept the inevitable or criticize how I look. Unfortunately, the media, fashion industry, and cosmetic industry have decided for women that aging is ugly. We can buy into this fact or ignore it.

The choice is ours to choose joy or succumb to the negative voices. The Bible says in I Samuel 16:7, "Do not consider his appearance or his height, for I have rejected him. The Lord does not look at the things people look at. People look at the outward appearance, but the Lord looks at the heart." (NIV) Ultimately, I believe, we want people to recognize our hearts.

People *will* judge us by our appearance. My hope is that we shine our light so brightly that people will *see* our true essence and move past initial judgments.

I share my story of losing weight and getting healthy, but the true benefits from this self-creation process was manifested through my surgery. If I had been heavier, I could have not had the procedure done through the laparoscope. The difference would have been days in the hospital and weeks of recovery as opposed to in and out of the hospital the same day. I started walking two days after my surgery. Two and a half weeks after the surgery, I returned to my strength training workouts. I had very little pain after the second day and eliminated the need for pain medication in three days.

The hospital kept me for an extra thirty minutes before my release because my heart rate was too low. Finally, they asked what type of physical activities I performed. When I told them about my twice-a-week weight training program, time spent on the treadmill, and walking my dog, they replied, "We're not used to seeing people like you." I was very happy for myself but saddened by the comment to know that the majority of people don't take time to care for their health.

As a result of becoming healthier, I watched my cholesterol; triglycerides and blood pressure numbers reduce also. Doctors and health experts usually stress the importance of watching our weight and maintaining exercise. This surgery was my personal proof of its importance. That's why I wanted to share this final story with you.

I am always inspired by other people's stories. If you've been touched by *The Freedom to Eat*, I'd love to hear from you. Email me: support@jackietrottmann.com

Connect with me on social media:

(Please Follow and Like)
Facebook: https://www.facebook.comJackieTrottmannAuthor/
Pinterest: https://www.pinterest.com/jackietrottmann/
Instagram: https://www.intagram.com/jackietrottmann/
Linkedin: https://www.linkedin.com/in/jackietrottmann

To Freedom!

References

1. Beattie, Melody.
   Codependent No More.
   San Francisco: Harper & Row, 1987.
   How to stop controlling others and start caring for yourself
2. Pennebaker, James W. Ph.D.
   Opening Up – The Healing Power of Confiding in Others.
   New York: William Morrow and Company, Inc. Used by permission.
3. Scripture taken from the New King James Version®. Copyright © 1982 by Thomas Nelson, Inc. Used by permission.
4. Scripture quotations marked (NIV) are taken from the Holy Bible, New International Version®, NIV®. Copyright © 1973, 1978, 1984, 2011 by Biblica, Inc.™ Used by permission of Zondervan.

Resources

Gaining a Better Understanding of Yourself, Strengths, Personality, Spirituality

Strengths

StrengthsFinders® – <u>Now Discover Your Strengths</u> – Book and online: http://www.strengthsfinder.com ***Now Discover Your Strengths*** Buckingham, Marcus and Clifton, O. Donald, Ph.D. New York: Free Press, 2001. Discover the source of your strengths. *The Clear Channel workshop was based on this book. The book and workshop helped me to better understand myself and others in order to focus on my strengths. With each book, there is a code. This code gives you access to a website where you can go online and discover your top five strengths.*

Personality

Kiersey Temperament Sorter® – Free resource http://www.keirsey.com. *The Keirsey Temperament Sorter®-II (KTS®-II) is the most widely used personality instrument in the world. It is a powerful 70 question personality instrument that helps individuals discover their personality type. The KTS-II is based on Keirsey Temperament Theory™, published in the best selling books,* Please Understand Me® *and* Please Understand Me II, *by Dr. David Keirsey.*

Spirituality

The Riso-Hudson Enneagram Type Indicator https://tests.enneagraminstitute.com/test/1/code. The Enneagram Institute®, formed in 1997 by the late Don Richard Riso and by Russ Hudson, was created to further the research and development of the Enneagram, one of the most powerful and insightful tools for understanding ourselves and others. At its core, the Enneagram helps us to see ourselves at a deeper, more objective level and can be of invaluable assistance on our path to self-knowledge.

The Enneagram is used a lot by Spiritual Directors (persons trained to companion others on their spiritual paths). This resource is more suited to how we are wired spiritually. Cost is $12 and can be purchased through the link above.

Resources

Meditations

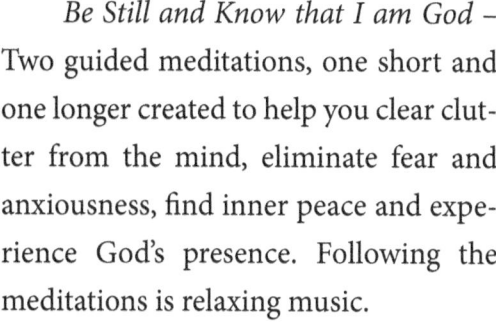

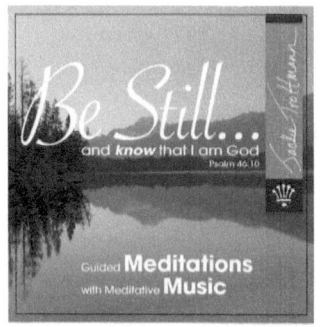

Be Still and Know that I am God – Two guided meditations, one short and one longer created to help you clear clutter from the mind, eliminate fear and anxiousness, find inner peace and experience God's presence. Following the meditations is relaxing music.

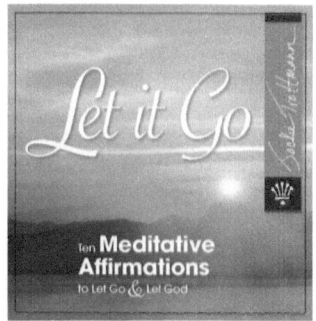

Let it Go - 10 Meditative Affirmations to Let Go and Let God – These meditative affirmations will help you to let go of past hurts, judgments, cravings, and limiting beliefs and embrace God's loving Spirit and unlimited potential within you. They were created to match the 10 Secrets and are the recorded prayers from each chapter.

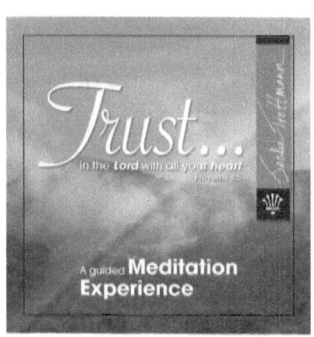

Trust – Why Trust is track 1 which goes into the importance of trust. There are two guided meditations. One is in the form of a prayer, the other is in the form of contemplative prayer. The latter leads you into a place of trust to meditate to music. Following the meditations is relaxing music.

Save when you purchase all three CDs. Be Still, Let it Go, Trust
You can listen to samples of each meditation,
visit JackieTrottmann.com.

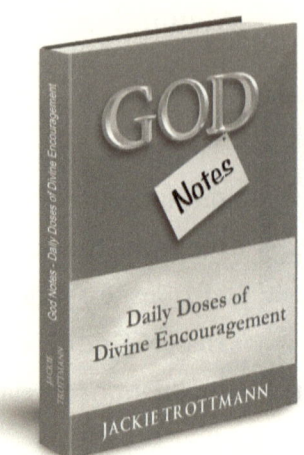

A Unique Daily Devotional

God Notes – Daily Doses of Divine Encouragement
One of the big deterrents to a meditation practice is that it takes time. Most people are time-poor.

They don't want to spend 10-20 minutes a day being still.

God Notes – Daily Doses of Divine Encouragement was created to offer people one simple word to meditate on throughout the day. The intention was: surely, people have time for one word!

I call God the God of surprises. I was surprised to find out that most people just open the book at random to see what word God has for them.

They like that there are no dates on the words because in other devotionals, if they skip a day, they feel guilty (which is not what daily devotionals are supposed to do!)

If you are looking for a simple book to add to your own Bible study and prayer, you will find simplicity in *God Notes*. It also makes a great gift to give encouragement to those you love.

To purchase go to: www.JackieTrottmann.com.

Encouragement through Email

Visit JackieTrottmann.com for more information.

Speaking and Workshops

Need a speaker for a book group, event, or workshop leader? Visit JackieTrottmann.com for more information.

Acknowledgments

Everyone needs someone to believe in them. My husband, Robert, always believed in me. Without his gift of telling me to quit my crazy job, I'd never be pursuing my dream of writing and creating. Thank you for believing in me and loving me unconditionally. I love you so much. You are a dream come true.

My greatest example of inspiration and living life on her terms was my mother, Bea Bumbicka. Music, primarily singing, was her passion. She made it her livelihood second to motherhood. Her purpose was singing and making people laugh. She did not hide her light under a bushel. It shown very brightly, lighting up the lives of people that she met. She was a good writer and always talked about writing a book but never did. The title would have been: And God Laughed.

Mom, I wish you had written that book. But your name at least made it into a book now! Thanks for being my biggest cheerleader growing up. And thank you for your strong faith and testimony of your close and personal relationship with God. I am grateful that you raised me to love God and to know what it's like to be loved by God, too. Your bright light is missed by so many.

Thank you to all who follow me through my blog, emails, social media, or through one or more of my meditations. Your vulnerability in sharing with me in return encourages and inspires me more than you will ever know.

Thank you, Caroline Ravelo, whose phone call inspired me to write *The Freedom to Eat* and is responsible for the start of my writing journey.

Thank you, Lynette Isaak, for your brilliant editing. You pointed out my blind spots and trimmed down the words that weren't necessary. You took my words and polished them to shine brightly.

Thank you, Jack Davis, for bringing *The Freedom to Eat* to life through your designing talent. Thank you, Cathy Davis, for encouraging me to do the illustrations and for helping me to navigate the complicated publishing waters which had been very murky and are now getting clear. I'd be lost without you!

Thank you to Rik Wilson, my trainer, mentor, friend. I can't believe that you are gone. Thank you for your support, brilliant training, your generosity, and being you. Your absence has left a hole in my heart that will never be filled.

Most of all, I thank God, whose unfathomable gifts of grace, peace, love, wholeness, creativity, and salvation are so freely given. You are reading these words because of the events and people nudged by God to bring the message onto the page.

About the Author

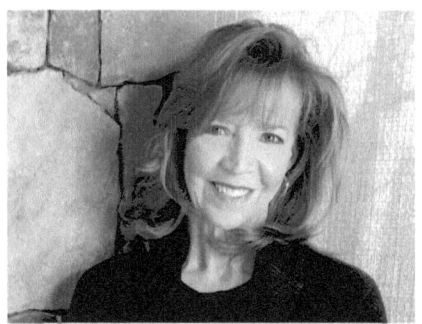

Jackie Trottmann left her corporate career behind to pursue God's call to share her personal experience of God's healing power and loving presence. Learning how to be still, let go, trust God, herself, and others, has been an ongoing spiritual practice. She teaches others how to do the same through her books, blog, meditation CDs, speaking, workshops, and other writing. This healing has led to living life with joy and flow. Jackie's greatest joy is found with pen and notebook in hand expressing God's latest inspiration, or behind a microphone recording the next project. Jackie shares her life and love of travel with husband, Robert, son Stephen, and lab, Wilson.

www.ingramcontent.com/pod-product-compliance
Lightning Source LLC
Chambersburg PA
CBHW020423010526
44118CB00010B/388